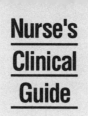

Nurse's Clinical Guide

DOSAGE CALCULATIONS

SECOND EDITION

D1567812

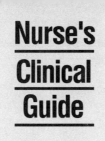

Nurse's
Clinical
Guide

DOSAGE CALCULATIONS

SECOND EDITION

Belle Erickson, RN,C, PhD
Assistant Professor
Villanova University, College of Nursing
Villanova, Pennsylvania

Catherine M.Todd, RN,C, EdD
Assistant Professor
Villanova University, College of Nursing
Villanova, Pennsylvania

Springhouse Corporation
Springhouse, Pennsylvania

STAFF

Executive Director, Editorial
Stanley Loeb

Senior Publisher, Trade and Textbooks
Minnie B. Rose, RN, BSN, MEd

Art Director
John Hubbard

Clinical Consultant
Susan Galea, RN, MSN

Associate Acquisitions Editors
Caroline Lemoine, Betsy K. Snyder

Editor
Nancy Priff

Copy Editor
Barbara Hodgson

Editorial Assistant
Louise Quinn

Designers
Stephanie Peters (associate art director), Elaine Ezrow, Laurie Mirijanian

Typography
Diane Paluba (manager), Elizabeth Bergman, Joyce Rossi Biletz, Phyllis Marron, Robin Mayer, Valerie L. Rosenberger

Manufacturing
Deborah Meiris (director), Anna Brindisi, Kate Davis, T.A. Landis

Some material in this book was adapted from *Dosage Calculations Manual*, 2nd ed., by Catherine M. Todd and Belle Erickson. © 1992 by Springhouse Corporation. Authorization to photocopy any items for internal or personal use, or the internal or personal use of specific clients, is granted by Springhouse Corporation for users registered with the Copyright Clearance Center (CCC) Transactional Reporting Service, provided that the base fee of $.75 per page is paid directly to CCC, 27 Congress St., Salem, MA 01970. For those organizations that have been granted a license by CCC, a separate system of payment has been arranged. The fee code for users of the Transactional Reporting Service is 0874343186/91 $00.00 + $.75.

Acknowledgments for photographs and equipment
p. 144 Lifecare PCA Plus II Infuser
Abbott Laboratories, Hospital Products Division, Abbott Park, Ill.

p. 146 Electronic volumetric controller and electronic infusion pump
IVAC Corporation, San Diego, Calif.

A member of the Reed Elsevier plc group

Library of Congress Cataloging-in-Publication Data

Erickson, Belle.
  Nurse's clinical guide, dosage calculations/Belle Erickson, Catherine M. Todd. — 2nd ed.
    p. cm.
  Rev. ed. of: Nurse's clinical guide, dosage calculation, ©1991.
  Includes bibliographical references and index.
  1. Pharmaceutical arithmetic. 2. Nursing. I. Todd, Catherine M. II. Erickson, Belle. Nurse's clinical guide, dosage calculations.
  III. Title. IV. Title: Dosage calculations.
    [DNLM: 1. Drugs — administration & dosage — nurses' instruction.
  2. Mathematics — nurses' instruction. QV 16 E68n 1994]
  RS57.E75 1994
  615.'14 — dc20
  DNLM/DLC   94-3506
  ISBN 0-87434-703-3   CIP

CONTENTS

CONTENTS (continued)

PREFACE

Administering medications safely is one of the most important aspects of nursing practice. It demands adherence to the classic safeguards—the five "rights" of medication administration: right drug, right dose, right route, right time, and right patient. Furthermore, to administer the right dose, the nurse not only must confirm information but also in many cases must be skilled in computation and reconstitution.

Nurse's Clinical Guide to Dosage Calculations, Second Edition, provides the information you need to prepare and administer medications properly and confidently. For most calculations, the text presents several mathematical approaches and uses examples to explore each, thus enabling you to choose the one with which you feel most comfortable. Numerous problems and their solutions are built around patient situations, which demonstrate how you can apply theoretical calculation skills to actual clinical practice. These also prepare you for practice problems (with answers) that conclude each chapter.

Throughout the text, a wide variety of tables, new illustrations, and photographs of equipment and the latest drug labels familiarize you with vital information related to accurate dosage calculations and safe drug administration. As an added feature, the text includes information related to specialty areas—such as obstetrics, pediatrics, critical care, oncology, and geriatrics—so you'll feel equipped to perform dosage calculations accurately in many settings.

Chapter 1, Review of Mathematics, presents some of the mathematical skills needed to perform common dosage calculations and explains how to handle percentages as well as ratios and fractions in proportions. The chapter also contains a pre-test that assesses your ability to work with fractions and decimals.

Chapter 2, Systems of Drug Measurements, reviews the major systems of drug weights and measures, including the metric apothecaries', household, avoirdupois, and milliequivalent systems. It describes how to convert measurements within and among these systems and provides their common abbreviations.

Chapter 3, The Administration Process, provides an overview of the drug distribution system and details your responsibilities within it. Even if your institution uses the unit-dose system and you administer medications from single-dose packages, you still must know how to calculate dosages as a double check. The chapter also reviews how to read drug labels, interpret drug orders, and maintain records for all the medications you administer.

Chapter 4, Calculating Enteral Drug Dosages, discusses the computations you need when preparing medications absorbed via the intestinal route: tablets, capsules, elixirs, suspensions, and suppositories.

Chapter 5, Calculating Parenteral Drug Dosages, provides information about injectables, such as prepared liquids, reconstituted powders, and insulin. The chapter also reviews the calculations needed for I.V. fluid administration, total parenteral nutrition, infusion pumps, and patient-controlled analgesia.

Chapter 6, Solutions, Ointments, and Patches, describes the calculations for determining concentrations of enteral or topical solutions and provides administration guidelines for topical ointments and patches.

Chapter 7, Other Considerations, highlights the important factors you must keep in mind when performing dosage calculations for certain patients or certain drugs. The chapter reviews how to determine pediatric medication dosages and fluid needs, discusses chemotherapy dosages, and examines the special needs of geriatric patients and those of all ages who require individualized doses.

Two appendices—the first on converting temperatures and the second on performing dimensional analysis—summarize additional information that you are likely to want in clinical practice.

Nurse's Clinical Guide to Dosage Calculations, Second Edition, is the ideal resource for anyone who must prepare and administer medications. Professional nurses can use the text when a new type of calculation is required, when a calculation needs to be verified, or when a refresher is needed. Nursing students can use the text to learn and practice calculation skills they'll need for safe and accurate drug administration.

Belle Erickson, RN,C, PhD
Catherine M. Todd, RN,C, EdD

REVIEW
OF
MATHEMATICS

M odern nursing practice requires a sound background in basic mathematics, especially in calculating drug dosages. Although most institutions now use the unit-dose drug distribution system, which reduces the time you must spend calculating dosages, you must know how to perform accurate calculations to ensure that a patient receives correct dosages. Many medications are available only in fixed concentrations or strengths. The nurse must be able to use fractions, decimals, and ratio and fraction proportions to calculate the appropriate dosage for a patient. (See *The unit-dose system.*)

This chapter briefly reviews some of the mathematical skills required for most common dosage calculations and explains how to handle percentages as well as ratios and fractions in propor-

---

THE UNIT-DOSE SYSTEM

For many years, the nurse spent a great deal of time calculating doses and pouring medications, and these time-consuming tasks took away from the more important aspects of the medication administration process. In the last decade, the use of the unit-dose drug distribution system has reduced this burden and has provided more time for evaluating patient responses to medications and teaching patients about their drug regimens.

This timesaving system provides you with the exact dose of medication needed for each patient. In the unit-dose system, the pharmacist computes the number of tablets or the volume of liquid required and prepares the proper dose for administration. You, however, must still be able to perform the necessary calculations for measuring correct doses, because some institutions do not have unit-dose systems and others do not have systems that operate 24 hours a day.

tions. It also provides examples to demonstrate these mathematical skills, and practice problems to allow you to develop and improve these skills.

Before you read the rest of this text, take the following pretest to assess your ability to work with fractions and decimals. You will need a good foundation in basic mathematics to understand and perform the computations presented in this book. If you require additional practice, consult a basic mathematics textbook.

PRE-TEST

This pre-test assesses your knowledge of basic mathematical concepts and your ability to solve common arithmetic problems. To check your answers, see pages 11 and 12.

1. In the fraction $\frac{2}{7}$, which number is the numerator and which is the denominator?

2. Of the fractions $\frac{1}{2}$, $\frac{5}{7}$, and $\frac{7}{6}$, which is the improper fraction?

3. Reduce the following fractions to their lowest terms.
a) $\frac{4}{6}$
b) $\frac{25}{100}$
c) $\frac{6}{18}$

4. Of the numbers 2, 5, and 9, which one is not a prime factor?

5. For the fractions $\frac{1}{5}$, $\frac{1}{6}$, and $\frac{1}{8}$, what is the lowest common denominator?

6. Add the following sets of fractions.
a) $\frac{2}{3} + \frac{1}{6} + \frac{2}{5}$
b) $\frac{1}{10} + \frac{1}{15} + \frac{1}{6}$
c) $\frac{1}{7} + \frac{1}{8} + \frac{2}{9}$

7. Subtract the following fractions.
a) $\frac{7}{8} - \frac{3}{4}$
b) $\frac{2}{3} - \frac{1}{4}$
c) $\frac{1}{6} - \frac{1}{8}$

8. Multiply the following fractions.
a) $\frac{2}{7} \times \frac{8}{9}$
b) $1\frac{1}{2} \times \frac{7}{8}$
c) $3\frac{1}{4} \times 5\frac{1}{8}$

9. Simplify the following complex fractions.

a) $\dfrac{^6/_7}{^7/_8}$

b) $\dfrac{^2/_3}{^3/_7}$

c) $\dfrac{^5/_6}{^1/_3}$

10. Divide the following fractions.

a) $1\frac{1}{2} \div \frac{2}{3}$

b) $\frac{7}{8} \div \frac{4}{5}$

c) $\frac{4}{7} \div \frac{5}{6}$

11. For each of the following decimals, what number is in the hundredths place?

a) 3.124

b) 0.1057

c) 12.879

12. Round off the following decimals to the nearest tenth.

a) 8.245

b) 10.2367

c) 0.252

13. Add the following decimals.

a) 0.234 + 1.1

b) 7.3 + 4.578 + 9.07

c) 0.456 + 0.06 + 8.970

14. Subtract the following decimals.

a) 10.005 − 0.05

b) 0.75 − 0.025

c) 1.5 − 0.005

15. Multiply the following decimals.

a) 4.5 × 0.025

b) 2.1 × 10.003

c) 9.1 × 0.2

REVIEW OF PERCENTAGES

Percentages represent an alternate way to express fractions and numerical relationships. A common term, *percentage* means any quantity stated as the proportion per hundred and is expressed with a % sign, which means "for every hundred." This symbol may be used with a whole number (10%), a mixed number (12½%), a decimal number (0.9%), or a fraction number (¼%). You should be able to convert freely from percentages to decimals and common fractions, and from these decimals and fractions to percentages.

Converting a percentage to a decimal

To change a percentage to a decimal, you can multiply by 0.01. For example, 72% would be: $72 \times 0.01 = 0.72$. Or you can use an even simpler conversion technique. Remove the percent sign and move the decimal point two places to the left, as shown below:

Convert 15% to a decimal.

Remove the percent sign.

15

Move the decimal point two places to the left to obtain the decimal.

0.15

Convert 6.25% to a decimal.

Remove the percent sign.

6.25

Move the decimal point two places to the left to obtain the decimal.

0.0625

Converting a decimal to a percentage

To change a decimal to a percentage, reverse the process. Move the decimal point two places to the right and add a percent sign, as shown below:

Convert 0.33 to a percentage.

Move the decimal point two places to the right.

33

Add a percent sign to obtain the percentage.

33%

Convert 0.125 to a percentage.

Move the decimal point two places to the right.

12.5

Add a percent sign to obtain the percentage.

12.5%

Converting a common fraction to a percentage

You can convert any common fraction to a percentage using two simple steps. First, convert the fraction to a decimal by dividing the numerator by the denominator. (A hand-held calculator makes this part of the conversion particularly easy.) Then, move the decimal point two places to the right, round off to the appropriate number of places (if necessary), and add the percent sign, as shown below:

Convert ⅜ to a percentage.
   Convert ⅜ to a decimal by dividing 8 into 3.

$$0.375$$

   Convert the decimal to a percentage by moving the decimal point two places to the right and adding the % sign.

$$37.5\%$$

Convert ⅔ to a percentage.
   Convert ⅔ to a decimal by dividing 3 into 2. (Round off to two decimal places.)

$$0.666 = 0.67$$

   Convert the decimal to a percentage by moving the decimal point two places to the right and adding the % sign.

$$67\%$$

Converting a percentage to a common fraction

To convert a percentage to a common fraction, follow these three steps. First, change the percentage to a decimal by removing the percent sign and moving the decimal point two places to the left. Second, convert the decimal to a common fraction with the appropriate denominator. Third, reduce the fraction to its lowest terms. This three-step process is shown below:

Convert 37.5% to a common fraction.
   Convert 37.5% to a decimal by removing the % sign and moving the decimal point two places to the left.

$$0.375$$

   Convert the decimal to a common fraction by using 1,000 as the denominator because there are three decimal places.

$$375/1{,}000$$

   Reduce the common fraction to the lowest terms.

$$3/8$$

Solving percentage problems

When solving a percentage problem to find the percent of a number, remember to change the percentage to a decimal and to use the word *of* to mean *multiply*. When solving a percentage problem to find the percent one number is of another, use *of* to mean *divide*. When solving a percentage problem to find the number that another number is the percentage of, change the percentage to a decimal and divide this into the number. Problems of this type may also be set up as a ratio proportion with one unknown, then solved for X. (See "Using ratios in proportions," page 8.) These key points make the solving of percentage problems much easier, as shown below:

What is 15% of 300?

Convert 15% to a decimal by moving the decimal point two places to the left and removing the percent sign.

$$0.15$$

Multiply to solve for the percent.

$$\begin{array}{r} 0.15 \\ \times \quad 300 \\ \hline 45 \end{array}$$

25 is what percent of 200?

Rewrite the problem to divide 25 by 200.

$$200\overline{)\,25.00\,}^{\,0.125}$$

Move the decimal point in the answer (quotient) two plac to the right.

$$0.125 = 12.5$$

Add the percent sign.

$$12.5\%$$

What percent of 16 is 8?

Rewrite the problem to divide 8 by 16.

$$16\overline{)\,8.00\,}^{\,0.50}$$

Move the decimal point two places to the right.

$$0.50 = 50$$

Add the percent sign.

$$50\%$$

The answer may also include a common fraction: 2 is what percent of 9?

Rewrite to divide 2 by 9, leaving the remainder after two places as a common fraction.

$$\frac{0.22\%}{9\ \overline{\smash{)}\ 2.00}}$$

Move the decimal point in the answer (quotient) two places to the right.

$$0.22\% = 22\%$$

Add the percent sign.

$$22\%\%$$

70% of what number is 42?

Convert 70% to a decimal by removing the percent sign and moving the decimal point two places to the left.

$$70\% = 0.70$$

Divide the decimal into the number (divide the number by the decimal).

$$070\ \overline{\smash{)}\ 4200}\ \ \ \frac{60.}{}$$

REVIEW OF RATIOS AND FRACTIONS IN PROPORTIONS

A *ratio* and a *fraction* are numerical ways to compare items. If a hospital hires three ancillary workers for every professional hired, then the ratio of ancillary workers to professionals is 3 to 1. This can be written as the ratio 3:1 or as the fraction ³⁄₁. In a ratio or fraction, you must pay attention to which item is mentioned first. For example, the ratio of ancillary workers to professionals is 3 to 1, but the ratio of professionals to ancillary workers is 1 to 3, which can be written as 1:3 or ⅓.

A *proportion* is a set of two equal ratios or fractions. For example, if the above ratio of ancillary workers to professionals is 3:1, then this would mean six ancillary workers for every two professionals. These proportions could be written as shown below:

$$3:1 :: 6:2$$
or
$$\frac{3}{1} = \frac{6}{2}$$

Using ratios in proportions

When a proportion is written with a double colon separating the ratios, as in 3:1 :: 6:2, the proportion's outer numbers (3 and 2) are the *extremes,* and its inner numbers (1 and 6) are the *means.* In such a proportion, the product of the means equals the product of the extremes. In this case, $1 \times 6 = 3 \times 2$. This principle lets you solve for any one of four unknown parts in a proportion, as shown below:

Solve for X in this proportion.

$$3:8 :: 6:X$$

Rewrite the problem to multiply the means and the extremes.

$$3 \times X = 8 \times 6$$

Obtain the products of the means and extremes in an equation.

$$3X = 48$$

Solve for X by dividing both sides by 3.

$$\frac{3X}{3} = \frac{48}{3}$$

Find X.

$$X = 16$$

Restate the proportion in ratios.

$$3:8 :: 6:16$$

Using fractions in proportions

In a fractionally expressed proportion, *cross products* are equal. In other words, the numerator on the equation's left side multiplied by the denominator on the equation's right side equals the denominator on the equation's left side multiplied by the numerator on the equation's right side. The cross products of a proportion allow you to solve for any one of four unknown parts in the proportion, as shown below:

Solve for X in this proportion.

$$\frac{5}{2} = \frac{X}{4}$$

Rewrite the problem to multiply the cross products.

$$2 \times X = 5 \times 4$$

Obtain the cross products.

$$2X = 20$$

Solve for X by dividing both sides by 2.

$$\frac{2X}{2} = \frac{20}{2}$$

Find X.

$$X = 10$$

Restate the proportion in fractions.

$$\frac{5}{2} = \frac{10}{4}$$

Setting up proportions

When setting up a proportion, place the known ratio on one side of the double colon and the ratio with the unknown on the other side, making certain that the similar parts of each ratio are in the same position relative to the colon. Thus, if you know how much salt (½ tsp) is added to an 8-oz cup of water to make a particular solution, but you wish to make up a quart of solution, the proportion would be written as:

½ tsp salt : 8 oz water :: X tsp salt : 32 oz (1 qt) water

$$8X = \frac{1}{2} \times 32$$
$$8X = 16$$
$$\frac{8X}{8} = \frac{16}{8}$$
$$X = 2 \text{ tsp salt}$$

If setting up the proportion fractionally, observe the same rule in placing like parts of the ratios.

$$\frac{\frac{1}{2} \text{ tsp salt}}{8 \text{ oz water}} = \frac{X \text{ tsp salt}}{32 \text{ oz water}}$$
$$8X = 16$$
$$X = 2 \text{ tsp salt}$$

PRACTICE PROBLEMS

Percentages
The answers to these problems follow on page 12.

1. What is 25% of 200?

2. 0.125 is what percent of 0.25?

3. What is 11.3% of 25?

4. ¼ is what percent of ½?

5. What is 5% of 1,000?

6. 250 is what percent of 1,000?

7. What is 0.9% of 1,000?

8. 30 is what percent of 50?

9. What is 0.45% of 500?

10. 1⅓ is what percent of 2?

Proportions

Solve for X in the following proportions. Check your answers against those on page 12.

1. X:4 :: 3:5

2. X:100 :: 100:1,000

3. ¼:1 :: ½:X

4. X:0.25 :: 0.5:1

5. 3:10 :: 12:X

6. 5:6 :: 7:X

7. 3:X :: 12:36

8. 7:1 :: 49:X

9. 2.2:3.5 :: 1:X

10. $\dfrac{X}{55} = \dfrac{1}{2.2}$

11. $\dfrac{X}{75} = \dfrac{0.5}{50}$

12. $\dfrac{X}{100} = \dfrac{5}{125}$

13. $\dfrac{½}{0.5} = \dfrac{¼}{X}$

14. $\dfrac{80}{10} = \dfrac{60}{X}$

15. $\dfrac{6}{7} = \dfrac{24}{X}$

16. $\dfrac{X}{7} = \dfrac{5}{35}$

ANSWERS TO PRE-TEST

1. 2 is the numerator, 7 is the denominator

2. $7/6$ is the improper fraction

3. a) $2/3$
   b) $1/4$
   c) $1/3$

4. 9 is not a prime factor, as it is divisible by 3

5. 120 is the lowest common denominator
   ($1/5 = 24/120$, $1/6 = 20/120$, $1/8 = 15/120$)

6. a) $2/3 + 1/6 + 2/5 = 20/30 + 5/30 + 12/30 = 37/30 = 1\,7/30$
   b) $1/10 + 1/15 + 1/6 = 3/30 + 2/30 + 5/30 = 10/30 = 1/3$
   c) $1/7 + 1/8 + 2/9 = 72/504 + 63/504 + 112/504 = 247/504$

7. a) $7/8 - 3/4 = 7/8 - 6/8 = 1/8$
   b) $2/3 - 1/4 = 8/12 - 3/12 = 5/12$
   c) $1/6 - 1/8 = 4/24 - 3/24 = 1/24$

8. a) $2/7 \times 8/9 = 16/63$
   b) $1\frac{1}{2} \times 7/8 = 3/2 \times 7/8 = 21/16 = 1\,5/16$
   c) $3\frac{1}{4} \times 5\frac{1}{8} = 13/4 \times 41/8 = 533/32 = 16\,21/32$

9. a) $6/7 \times 8/7 = 48/49$
   b) $2/3 \times 7/3 = 14/9 = 1\,5/9$
   c) $5/6 \times 3/1 = 15/6 = 2\,3/6 = 2\frac{1}{2}$

10. a) $1\frac{1}{2} \div 2/3 = 3/2 \times 3/2 = 9/4 = 2\frac{1}{4}$
    b) $7/8 \div 4/5 = 7/8 \times 5/4 = 35/32 = 1\,3/32$
    c) $4/7 \div 5/6 = 4/7 \times 6/5 = 24/35$

11. a) 2
    b) 0
    c) 7

12. a) 8.2
    b) 10.2
    c) 0.3

13. a)
$$\begin{array}{r} 0.234 \\ +\ 1.100 \\ \hline 1.334 \end{array}$$
b)
$$\begin{array}{r} 7.300 \\ 4.578 \\ +\ 9.070 \\ \hline 20.948 \end{array}$$
c)
$$\begin{array}{r} 0.456 \\ 0.060 \\ +\ 8.970 \\ \hline 9.486 \end{array}$$

14. a)
$$\begin{array}{r} 10.005 \\ -\ 0.050 \\ \hline 9.955 \end{array}$$
b)
$$\begin{array}{r} 0.750 \\ -\ 0.025 \\ \hline 0.725 \end{array}$$
c)
$$\begin{array}{r} 1.500 \\ -\ 0.005 \\ \hline 1.495 \end{array}$$

15. a)
```
        0.025
    ×     4.5
        125
        100
      0.1125
```
b)
```
       10.003
    ×      2.1
       10003
       20006
      21.0063
```
c)
```
          9.1
    ×     0.2
         1.82
```

ANSWERS TO PRACTICE PROBLEMS

Percentages

1. 50
2. 50%
3. 2.825 = 2.8
4. 50%
5. 50
6. 25%
7. 9
8. 60%
9. 2.25
10. 66.66 = 66.7

Proportions

1. X = 2.4
2. X = 10
3. X = 2
4. X = 0.125
5. X = 40
6. X = 8⅖ = 8.4
7. X = 9
8. X = 7
9. X = 1.59 = 1.6
10. X = 25
11. X = 0.75
12. X = 4
13. X = 0.25
14. X = 7.5
15. X = 28
16. X = 1

2

SYSTEMS OF DRUG MEASUREMENTS

This chapter examines the major systems of drug weights and measures, including the metric, apothecaries', household, avoirdupois, unit, and milliequivalent systems. It describes equivalent measures among these systems and presents their common abbreviations.

METRIC SYSTEM

In high school and in college science courses, students usually learn the metric system, the measurement system used by most nations. Because the metric system is based on powers of 10, it offers several advantages over other measurement systems: it eliminates common fractions, simplifies calculation of larger or smaller units, and simplifies calculation of drug dosages.

Metric terms

The first step in understanding the metric system is to become familiar with its three basic units of measurement: the meter, liter, and gram.

The *meter* (m) is the basic unit of length. The *liter* (L) is the basic unit of volume, representing one tenth of a cubic meter. The *gram* (G, Gm, or GM) is the basic unit of weight, representing the weight of one cubic centimeter of water at 4° C. The preferred abbreviation for gram is "G." The abbreviations "gm" and "g" should not be used; they can be easily confused with "gr" (grain) when handwritten, which could lead to dangerous errors. "GM" is an old abbreviation for gram that still may be used by some physicians. (See *Metric measurement devices*, page 14, for an illustration.) Besides the three basic units of measurement, the

METRIC MEASUREMENT DEVICES

The three basic units in the metric system—the meter, liter, and gram—must be measured with different devices. A meterstick, which resembles a yardstick, is used to measure length. A metric graduate can be used to measure volume in liters. A set of metric weights can be used to measure weight in grams. An enclosed chamber is required to measure a volume of gas, such as the cylinder formed by the barrel of a syringe.

METRIC GRADUATES

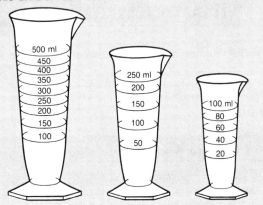

SET OF METRIC WEIGHTS

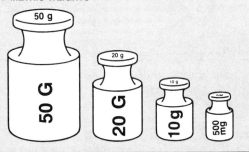

PORTION OF METERSTICK (with centimeters and inches)

metric system includes other units that are multiples of the basic units. Each of these units has a prefix indicating its relationship to the basic unit and an abbreviation for ease of notation. For example, the most common subdivision of the gram is the *milli*gram (mg), which represents one thousandth or 0.001 of a gram. The most common multiple of a gram is the *kilo*gram (kg), which is 1,000 times greater than the gram. These prefixes and others apply to meters, liters, and grams and can be used to express units of measure ranging from kilometers (km) to nanograms (ng) to deciliters (dl). (See *Metric system prefixes, abbreviations, and values,* page 16, for a listing.)

The metric system also includes one unusual unit of volume, the cubic centimeter (cc). Because the cubic centimeter occupies the same space as one milliliter of liquid, these two units of volume are considered equal and are frequently used interchangeably. (Technically, however, cubic centimeters refer to gas volume and milliliters refer to liquid volume.)

Metric conversions

Because the metric system has a decimal basis, conversions between units of measure are fairly easy. To convert a smaller unit to a larger one, move the decimal point to the left or divide by the appropriate multiple of 10. To convert a larger unit to a smaller one, move the decimal point to the right or multiply by the appropriate multiple of 10.

For example, to convert from grams to milligrams (one thousandth of a gram), you would multiply by 1,000, or move the decimal three places to the right. Likewise, to convert from milligrams to grams, you would divide by 1,000, or move the decimal three places to the left.

The following scale and examples illustrate the process.

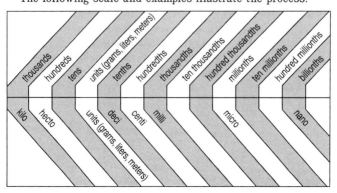

METRIC SYSTEM PREFIXES, ABBREVIATIONS, AND VALUES

In the metric system, the addition of a prefix to one of the basic units of measure indicates a multiple or subdivision of that unit. To abbreviate these units of measure, place the prefix abbreviation before the abbreviation L (for liter) or G (for gram). For example, abbreviate kilogram as kg and milliliter as ml.

PREFIX	ABBREVIATION	MULTIPLES AND SUBDIVISIONS (FRACTIONS)
kilo	k	1,000
hecto	h	100
deka	dk	10
deci	d	0.1 (1/10th)
centi	c	0.01 (1/100th)
milli	m	0.001 (1/1,000th)
micro	mc	0.000001 (1/1,000,000th)
nano	n	0.000000001 (1/1,000,000,000th)

To convert 5 m to kilometers, first count the number of places to the right or left of "meter" to reach "kilo" on the scale. Because a kilo is three decimal places to the left of a meter (1,000 times larger), you would move the decimal point to the left, indicating that 5 m equal 0.005 km. Remember to place a zero in front of the decimal point.

To convert 50 mg to micrograms (mcg), locate "milli" and "micro" on the scale. The Greek symbol µg sometimes is used for microgram but is not recommended because it can be misinterpreted to mean mg. Because a microgram is three decimal places to the right of milligram, or 1,000 times smaller, you would move the decimal point to the right, indicating that 50 mg equal 50,000 mcg.

To convert 250 centiliters (cl) to liters, find these units on the scale. Because a liter is two places to the left of a centiliter, or 100 times larger, you would move the decimal point two places to the left, indicating that 250 cl equal 2.5 L.

To speed metric conversions, you can memorize the equivalents of commonly used measures. (See *Metric measures,* page 18, for a listing.)

Patient situations

1. A baby weighs 4.72 kg. What is the baby's weight in grams?

■ Knowing that 1 kg is equal to 1,000 G, set up the following equation:

$$X \text{ G} = 4.72 \text{ kg} \times 1,000 \text{ G/kg}$$

■ Solving for X, you find the baby weighs 4,720 G.

2. A patient received 0.5 L of intravenous fluid. How many milliliters did the patient receive?

First, find "liter" and then "milli" on the metric conversion scale. Because "milli" is located three places to the right of "liter," move the decimal point three places to the right, indicating that 0.5 L is equal to 500 ml.

Metric mathematics

Once you can convert from one metric unit to another, you can solve basic arithmetic problems in metric units. To add, subtract, multiply, or divide different metric units, you first must convert all quantities to the same metric unit. Unless the problem calls for an answer in a particular unit, you may use whichever common unit is easiest to work with. Then you can perform the arithmetic operation, as shown in the following examples.

To add 1 kg, 250 mg, and 7.5 G and express the total in grams, convert all units to grams and add:

$$
\begin{array}{rl}
1 \text{ kg} = & 1,000.0 \text{ G} \\
250 \text{ mg} = & 0.250 \text{ G} \\
7.5 \text{ G} = & \underline{+ \quad 7.5 \text{ G}} \\
\text{total} = & 1,007.75 \text{ G}
\end{array}
$$

To subtract 3.5 mg from 0.385 G and express the answer in micrograms, convert the units to micrograms and subtract:

$$
\begin{array}{rl}
0.385 \text{ G} = & 385,000 \text{ mcg} \\
3.5 \text{ mg} = & \underline{- \quad 3,500 \text{ mcg}} \\
\text{answer} = & 381,500 \text{ mcg}
\end{array}
$$

METRIC MEASURES

This table shows the equivalents of some commonly used metric measures. Several less commonly used measures, such as the hectogram, are included.

LIQUIDS
1 milliliter (ml) = 1 cubic centimeter (cc)
1,000 ml = 1 liter (L)
100 centiliters (cl) = 1 L
10 deciliters (dl) = 1 L
10 L = 1 dekaliter (dkl)
100 L = 1 hectoliter (hl)
1,000 L = 1 kiloliter (kl)

SOLIDS
1,000 micrograms (mcg) = 1 milligram (mg)
1,000 mg = 1 gram (G)
1,000 G = 1 kilogram (kg)
100 centigrams (cg) = 1 G
10 decigrams (dg) = 1 G
10 G = 1 dekagram (dkg)
100 G = 1 hectogram (hg)

Patient situation

A patient received 300 ml from a liter bag of intravenous fluid over the first shift, 275 ml over the second shift, and 225 ml over the third shift. How many milliliters of fluid remain in the I.V. bag?

■ First, determine how much fluid the patient received. To do this, add:

$$
\begin{array}{r}
300 \text{ ml} \\
275 \text{ ml} \\
+\ 225 \text{ ml} \\
\hline
X \text{ ml}
\end{array}
$$

■ Solving for X, you find that the patient has received 800 ml of fluid.

■ Next, you need to convert all of the measures to the same units. Either 1 L must be converted to milliliters, or 800 ml must be converted to liters. Since the number of milliliters remaining needs to be determined, you decide to convert 1 L to milliliters. Using the equivalency chart, you find that 1 L is equal to 1,000 ml.

■ Compute the amount of fluid remaining by subtracting:

$$
\begin{array}{r}
1,000 \text{ ml} \\
- 800 \text{ ml} \\
\hline
\text{X ml}
\end{array}
$$

■ Solving for X, you find that there should be 200 ml of fluid remaining in the patient's I.V. bag.

APOTHECARIES', HOUSEHOLD, AND OTHER SYSTEMS

Besides the metric system, you may use the apothecaries', household, unit, and milliequivalent systems when preparing and administering drugs. You also may use the avoirdupois system for requisitioning pharmaceutical products and for weighing patients. This section will show you how to use these measurement systems appropriately and will explain equivalent measures among various systems.

Apothecaries' system

Physicians and pharmacists used the apothecaries' system of measurement before the metric system. After the metric system was introduced, however, use of the older system began to decline. Although the apothecaries' system is being phased out, it still is being used on a very limited basis. Therefore, you may see prescriptions and bottle labels that use it.

The apothecaries' system traditionally uses Roman numerals and places the unit of measurement before the Roman numerals. For example, *5 grains* would be written *grains v.* (Some physicians and other health care professionals do not follow this traditional convention. Instead, they express apothecaries' system dosages in Arabic numbers followed by units of measurement, such as *5 grains.*)

Roman numerals

A physician who writes prescriptions in the apothecaries' system usually expresses quantities of drugs or ingredients with Roman numerals. The following letters, when used as Roman numerals, indicate these numeric values:

$\overline{ss}$ = ½	L = 50
I = 1	C = 100
V = 5	D = 500
X = 10	M = 1,000

In pharmacologic applications, Roman numerals ss (an abbreviation of the Latin word *semis,* meaning half) through X usually are written in lower case: $\overline{ss}$, i, v, and x, often with a line above, as in $\overline{ss}$. The dot over the i helps to clarify this symbol as a one and prevents mistaking $\overline{iii}$ for $\overline{iv}$. Fractions of less than one-half ($\overline{ss}$) are written as common fractions using Arabic numbers.

Units of measurement

With the metric system, you can measure length in meters, volume in liters, and weight in grams. With the apothecaries' system, however, you can measure only volume and weight. In this system, the basic unit for measuring liquid volume is the minim (M_x) and that for measuring solid weight is the grain (gr). To visualize these standards, remember that a minim is about the size of a drop of water, which weighs about the same as a grain of wheat. The following mathematical statement sums up this relationship:

$$1 \text{ drop} \approx 1 \text{ minim } (M_x) \approx 1 \text{ grain (gr)}.$$

Remember, however, that these are only approximate equivalents. For example, the size of an actual drop varies with the density and viscosity of the liquid (if other than water) and with the size and configuration of the dropper.

Other units of measure in the apothecaries' system build on these basic units. (See *Apothecaries' measures,* page 22, for a complete listing.) Many of these units also are used as common household measures. A discussion of the relationship between apothecaries', household, and metric measures appears later in this chapter.

Patient situations

1. Part of a physician's order is written *Give Tylenol gr x̄ for Temp. > 100° F.* How many grains of the medication must you administer?

You need to convert gr x̄ from Roman numerals to Arabic. Gr represents grains, and x in Roman numerals is equal to 10 in Arabic numbers.

Thus, gr x̄ = grains 10 = 10 grains of Tylenol.

2. You note that a patient will require five 4-oz doses of a medication. The drug is available only in 1-pt bottles. How many bottles of the drug will the patient need?

■ First, you must determine the total amount of medication the patient will need. The equation may be set up as:

$$\begin{array}{r} 4 \text{ oz} \\ \times\ 5 \text{ doses} \\ \hline X \text{ oz} \end{array}$$

■ Solving for X, you find that the patient will need 20 oz of the drug.

■ Using an equivalency table, you note that there are 16 oz in 1 pt. Set up the proportion:

$$\frac{X \text{ pt}}{20 \text{ oz}} = \frac{1 \text{ pt}}{16 \text{ oz}}$$

■ Solve for X:

$$X \text{ pt} \times 16 \text{ oz} = 20 \text{ oz} \times 1 \text{ pt}$$

$$X = \frac{20 \text{ pt}}{16}$$

$$X = 1.25 \text{ pt}$$

The patient will need 1.25 pt or 1¼ bottles of the medication. Thus, two bottles of the drug will be required.

You could approach the second part of this problem in another way:

$$\begin{array}{r} 20 \text{ oz (the total amount needed)} \\ -\ 16 \text{ oz (the amount provided by 1 bottle)} \\ \hline X \text{ oz} \end{array}$$

Solving for X, you would determine that, since 4 oz of medication will be needed after the first bottle is finished, the patient will require a second bottle.

APOTHECARIES' MEASURES

This table displays the relationships between measures of liquid volume and solid weight in the apothecaries' system.

LIQUID VOLUME
60 minims (M_x) = 1 dram (℥)
8 ℥ = 1 ounce (℥)
16 (℥) = 1 pint (pt)
2 pt = 1 quart (qt)
4 qt = 1 gallon (gal)
SOLID WEIGHT
60 grains (gr) = 1 ℥
8 ℥ = 1 ℥
12 ℥ = 1 pound (lb)

Household system

Many of the units of liquid measure in the apothecaries' system are identical to those used in the household system of measurement. Because all droppers, teaspoons, tablespoons, and glasses are not alike, the household system of liquid measurement can be used for approximate measures only. In the hospital setting, you should not use the household system to measure medications. You should use the apothecaries' or metric system.

Most people in the United States are familiar with the household system of weights and measures. In most cases, food products, recipes, over-the-counter drugs, and home remedies use the household system. Although the household system is of limited use in the hospital setting, the home health nurse needs to be familiar with it because the patient may use this measurement system at home and is likely to be the most comfortable with it.

HOUSEHOLD MEASURES

This table shows the equivalents of the most commonly used household measures, which are used to measure liquid volume. Note: The abbreviations "t" (teaspoon) and "T" (tablespoon) should be avoided because they carry a high potential for error when written quickly. Always clarify a prescription that includes these symbols.

LIQUIDS
60 drops (gtt) = 1 teaspoon (tsp)
3 tsp = 1 tablespoon (Tbs)
2 Tbs = 1 ounce (oz)
8 oz = 1 cup (c)
16 oz (2 c) = 1 pint (pt)
2 pt = 1 quart (qt)
4 qt = 1 gallon (gal)

Most liquid medications are prescribed and dispensed in the metric system. To ensure the accuracy of dosages measured in the household system, you should teach the patient how to use devices that ensure more accurate drug measurement. (See *Household measures* and *Devices for administering liquid medications,* page 24, for further information.) You also can teach the patient conversions between household and metric measurements. (See "Equivalent measures among systems" on page 27.)

Avoirdupois system

You should be aware of the avoirdupois system because it is used for ordering and purchasing some pharmaceutical products and for weighing patients in clinical settings.

In the avoirdupois system, the solid measures or units of weight include grains, ounces (437.5 grains), and pounds (16 oz or 7,000 grains). Note that the apothecaries' pound equals 12 oz, but the avoirdupois pound equals 16 oz.

DEVICES FOR ADMINISTERING LIQUID MEDICATIONS

You should instruct the patient in using several devices that will help ensure accurate dosage measurements.

MEDICATION CUP
(calibrated in household, metric, and apothecaries' systems)
Teach the patient to set the cup on a counter and check the fluid measurement at eye level.

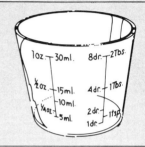

DROPPER
(calibrated in household or metric systems or in terms of medication strength or concentration)
Teach the patient to hold the dropper at eye level to check the fluid measurement.

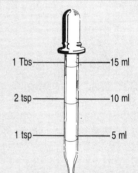

HOLLOW-HANDLE SPOON
(calibrated in teaspoons and tablespoons)
Teach the patient to check the dose after filling by holding the spoon upright at eye level. To administer, the patient tilts the spoon until the medication fills the bowl of the spoon and then places the spoon in his mouth.

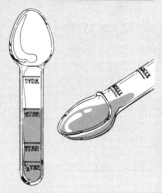

Unit system

Some drugs are not measured in the metric, apothecaries', or household systems. Rather, they are measured in units, such as United States Pharmacopeia (USP) units or International Units (IU). The most common drug measured in units (U) is insulin, which comes in 10-ml multidose vials of U-40 or U-100 strength. With this drug, the U refers to the number of units of insulin per milliliter. For example, 1 ml of U-40 insulin contains 40 units; 1 ml of U-100 insulin contains 100 units. Use of U-40 insulin has declined in recent years; the U-100 strength, which is based on metric measurement, makes measurement in a standard syringe easier. (See Chapter 5, Calculating Parenteral Drug Dosages.)

Other drugs are also measured in units. For example, the anticoagulant heparin is available in liquid forms that contain 10 to 20,000 units/ml for parenteral use. Bacitracin, an antibiotic, is available in a topical form that contains 50 units/ml. Penicillins G and V are available in different forms that contain 400,000 units/ml (approximately equal to 250 mg) or 800,000 units/ml (approximately equal to 500 mg). The hormone calcitonin is measured in IU, as are the fat-soluble vitamins A, D, and E. Some forms of vitamins A and D also are measured in USP units.

To calculate the dose to be administered when the medication is available in units, use the following proportion:

$$\frac{\text{amount of drug (ml)}}{\text{dose of drug required (units)}} = \frac{1 \text{ ml}}{\text{drug available (units)}}$$

Patient situations

1. A patient requires 24 units of insulin daily. How many milliliters of U-100 insulin should be given?

▪ First, identify the insulin available (100 units/ml) and the dose of insulin required (24 units). Then, set up the proportion:

$$\frac{X \text{ ml}}{24 \text{ units}} = \frac{1 \text{ ml}}{100 \text{ units}}$$

▪ Solve for X:

$$X \text{ ml} \times 100 \text{ units} = 24 \text{ units} \times 1 \text{ ml}$$

$$X = \frac{24 \text{ ml}}{100}$$

$$X = 0.24 \text{ ml}$$

The patient should be given 0.24 ml of insulin.

2. If only U-40 insulin is available for a patient who needs 24 units daily, how many milliliters of insulin should be given?

■ Begin by identifying the insulin available (40 units/ml) and the dose of insulin required (24 units). Then, set up the proportion:

$$\frac{X \text{ ml}}{24 \text{ units}} = \frac{1 \text{ ml}}{40 \text{ units}}$$

■ Solve for X:

$$X \text{ ml} \times 40 \text{ units} = 24 \text{ units} \times 1 \text{ ml}$$

$$X = \frac{24 \text{ ml}}{40}$$

$$X = 0.6 \text{ ml}$$

The patient should be given 0.6 ml of insulin.

3. 400,000 units of Penicillin G is ordered for a patient. The pharmacy has run out of vials that contain 400,000 units/ml, so they send a vial labelled *Penicillin G 800,000 units/ml*. How many milliliters must be administered?

■ Set up the proportion:

$$\frac{X \text{ ml}}{400,000 \text{ units}} = \frac{1 \text{ ml}}{800,000 \text{ units}}$$

■ Solve for X:

$$X \text{ ml} \times 800,000 \text{ units} = 400,000 \text{ units} \times 1 \text{ ml}$$

$$X = \frac{400,000 \text{ ml}}{800,000}$$

$$X = 0.5 \text{ ml}$$

The patient should be given 0.5 ml of the Penicillin G solution.

Milliequivalent system

You will see electrolytes measured in milliequivalents (mEq). The drug manufacturers provide information about the number of metric units required to provide the prescribed number of milliequivalents. For example, the manufacturer's instructions may indicate that 1 ml equals 4 mEq.

A physician usually orders the electrolyte potassium chloride in milliequivalents. Potassium preparations for intravenous, oral, or other use are available as liquid (elixir and parenteral) and solid (powder and tablet) forms.

Patient situation

A patient who is receiving medications and feedings via a nasogastric tube is to receive 20 mEq of potassium chloride. You obtain the electrolyte in elixir form. The label states *Potassium Chloride, 30 mEq = 30 ml*. How many milliliters must be given to the patient?

▪ Set up the proportion:

$$\frac{X \text{ ml}}{20 \text{ mEq}} = \frac{30 \text{ ml}}{30 \text{ mEq}}$$

▪ Solve for X:

$$X \text{ ml} \times 30 \text{ mEq} = 20 \text{ mEq} \times 30 \text{ ml}$$

$$X = \frac{600 \text{ ml}}{30}$$

$$X = 20 \text{ ml}$$

More simply, you may have realized that if a solution contains 30 mEq in 30 ml, it contains 1 mEq/ml. Thus, if 20 mEq is needed, 20 ml should be given to the patient.

Equivalent measures among systems

In clinical practice, you may find that a physician's order for medication is written in one system of measurement whereas the medication is available in a different system. For example, the physician may order the medication in grains but the medication may be available in milligrams. To convert medication orders from one system to another, you must know the equivalent measures among systems of measurement.

Although references and charts that list equivalent measures among systems usually are available in the clinical setting, most nurses memorize the most frequently used equivalents. *Equivalent measures,* pages 28 and 29, lists the common equivalents among the metric, apothecaries', and household systems.

The plastic medication cup used for liquid preparations is also readily available in the clinical area, providing a quick reference for equivalents among measures in the metric, apothecaries', and household systems. Additionally, some syringes are labeled in both the metric and apothecaries' systems and can be used as a quick reference for liquid measures between these two systems.

EQUIVALENT MEASURES

The following shows some *approximate* liquid equivalents among the household, apothecaries', and metric systems.

Remember that an institution may acknowledge a particular set of equivalents as its official standard for exchange among systems. All health care professionals prescribing, dispensing, or administering drugs under such a purview should abide by the established protocol. If no protocol exists, use the equivalent that is easiest to manipulate in any given computation problem.

HOUSEHOLD	APOTHECARIES'	METRIC
1 drop (gtt)	1 minim (M_x)	0.06 milliliter (ml)
15* or 16 gtt	15* or 16 M_x	1 ml
1 teaspoon (tsp)	1 dram ʒ	4 or 5 ml
1 tablespoon (Tbs)	½ ʒ	15 or 16 ml
2 Tbs	1 ʒ	30* or 32 ml
1 cup (c)	8 ʒ	240* or 250 ml
1 pint (pt)	16 ʒ	480* or 500 ml
1 quart (qt)	32 ʒ	960 or 1,000* ml (1 liter)
1 gallon (gal)	128 ʒ	3,840 or 4,000* ml

The following shows some *approximate* solid equivalents among the avoirdupois, apothecaries', and metric systems.

AVOIRDUPOIS	APOTHECARIES'	METRIC
1 grain (gr)	1 grain (gr)	0.06* (or 0.065 gram [G])
15.4 gr	15 gr	1 G
1 ounce	480 gr	28.35 G
1 pound (lb)	1.33 lb	454 G
2.2 lb	2.7 lb	1 kg

*Indicates the most commonly used equivalent when more than one is listed here.

EQUIVALENT MEASURES (continued)

The following shows some *approximate* solid equivalents between the apothecaries' and metric systems.

APOTHECARIES'	METRIC
15 grains (gr) (¼ dram)	1 gram (G) (1,000 mg)
10 gr	0.6* G (600 mg)(or 0.65 G [650 mg])
7½ gr	0.5 G (500 mg)
5 gr	0.3* G (300 mg)(or 0.325 G [325 mg])
3 gr	0.2 G (200 mg)
1½ gr	0.1 G (100 mg)
1 gr	0.06* G (60 mg) (or 0.064 G [64 mg], or 0.065 G [65 mg])
¾ gr	0.05 G (50 mg)
½ gr	0.03* G (30 mg) (or 0.032 G [32 mg])
¼ gr	0.015* G (15 mg) (or 0.016 G [16 mg])
⅟₆₀ or ⅟₆₄ gr	0.001 G (1 mg)
⅟₁₀₀ gr	0.6 mg
⅟₁₂₀ gr	0.5 mg
⅟₁₅₀ gr	0.4 mg

*Indicates the most commonly used equivalent when more than one is listed here.

Patient situations

1. A patient has been taking 30 ml of a medication while hospitalized and is to continue taking this dose at home. The patient's medication cup at home is marked in ounces. How many ounces per dose should the patient take at home?

You know that 30 ml and 1 oz are equivalent measures. Thus, the patient should take 1 oz of the medication per dose at home.

To show the patient that the two measures are equivalent, you use a plastic medication cup labeled in milliliters and ounces.

2. A patient who must restrict daily fluid intake has been receiving 480 ml of fluid on each of the three daily food trays. The same fluid restriction is to continue at home, where available containers are marked in ounces, pints, and quarts. How much fluid is the patient permitted at each meal?

Use the following equivalent measures:

$$1 \text{ pt} = 16 \text{ oz} = 480 \text{ ml}$$
$$1 \text{ qt} = 32 \text{ oz}$$

Since the patient is permitted to have 480 ml of fluid at each meal, tell the patient this is equivalent to 1 pt, 16 oz, or ½ qt of fluid.

PRACTICE PROBLEMS

Metric terms and conversions
Answer the following questions to assess your progress. The answers to these problems follow on pages 37 to 39.

1. The measurement system based on grams, meters, and liters is the _____ system.

2. Of the following units of measure, _____,

_____, _____, and

_____ belong to the metric system.

ounce	milliliter	scruple
gram	inch	liter
teaspoon	centimeter	dram

3. In the metric system, the basic unit of length is the

_____ .

4. In the metric system, the gram is the basic unit used to measure _____ .

5. In the metric system, the basic unit used to measure volume is the _____ .

6. The abbreviation for gram is _____ .

7. The abbreviation for liter is _____ .

8. The abbreviation for microgram is _____ .

9. The abbreviation for milliliter is _____ .

10. The abbreviation for cubic centimeter is

_____ .

11. The millimeter equals _____ of a meter.

12. To convert milligrams to grams, move the decimal

point _____ places to the _____ .

13. To convert grams to milligrams, move the decimal

point _____ places to the _____ .

14. To convert kilograms to micrograms, move the dec-

imal point _____ places to the right.

15. 1,800 ml = _____ L.

16. 4,250 ml = _____ L.

17. 374 mcl = _____ ml.

18. 350 ml = _____ L.

19. 10 cc = _____ ml.

20. 1 L = _____ ml.

21. 1 ml = _____ L.

22. 58.5 L = _____ ml.

23. 150 cc = _____ ml.

24. 220 cc = _____ L.

25. 57,820 cc = _____ L.

26. 0.3 L = _____ ml.

27. 1 L = _____ dl.

28. 95 ml _____ cc.

29. 1 kg = _____ G.

30. 1 G = _____ mcg.

31. 1 G = _____ mg.

32. 52 G = _____ kg.

33. 6.2 G = _____ kg.

34. 732 G = _____ kg.

35. 17 G = _____ mg.

36. 0.17 G = _____ mg.

37. 0.47 G = _____ mg.

38. 286 G = _____ mg.

39. 160 mcg = _____ mg.

40. 1,970 mcg = _____ mg.

41. 119,200 mcg = _____ mg.

42. 600 mg = _____ G.

43. 50,000 mcg = _____ G.

44. 125 mcg = _____ mg.

45. 3,270 mcg = _____ mg.

46. 481,000 mcg = _____ G.

47. 305 G = _____ kg.

48. 1 mg = _____ mcg.

49. 1 mg = _____ ng.

50. 0.08 mcg = _____ ng.

51. 5.5 G = _____ mg.

52. 1 G = _____ ng.

53. 33 kg = _____ G.

54. 520 mg = _____ G.

55. 0.732 G = _____ mcg.

56. 0.47 G = _____ mg.

57. 25 mcg = _____ mg.

58. 0.083 mg = _____ mcg.

59. 300 ng = _____ mg.

60. 50 mg = _____ mcg.

Metric mathematics

These problems will test your ability to handle metric numbers. The answers to these practice problems follow on page 39.

1. 0.6 kg + 213 G + 360 mg + 12.4 G = _____ G.

2. 210 ml + 0.35 L + 65 cc + 2.6 L = _____ ml.

3. 1.4 G + 0.45 G + 180 mcg + 0.240 mg = _____ mg.

4. 2 G − 300 mg = _____ G.

5. 30 mg + 30 G + 215 mg + 2 kg + 454 G + 3,000 mg = _____ mg.

6. 1 L − 350 ml = _____ ml.

7. 4 kg + 44 G + 344 mg = _____ G.

8. 25 mg − 144 mcg = _____ mcg.

9. 0.25 G + 114 mg + 5,000 mcg + 0.03 kg = _____ mg.

10. 1,940 mg − 0.43 G = _____ G.

11. (0.05 G + 0.4 G) × ⅓ = _____ mg.

12. If you remove 20 mg, 235 mg, 0.855 G, and 35.5 mg of a drug from a container, a total of _____ G will have been removed.

13. If you remove 0.5 L and 500 ml of a drug from a 4-L container, _____ L will be left.

14. After you remove 320 ml, 15 ml, 130 ml, and 1.2 L from a 2-L bottle, _____ ml will be left.

15. If you divide 3.2 G of a drug into eight equal doses, each dose will weigh _____ mg.

16. If 15 tablets of an investigational drug weigh a total of 0.825 G, each tablet must weigh _____ mg.

17. If you administer 250 mg of cefazolin sodium (Ancef) from a 1-G vial, _____ mg will be left.

18. If one phenobarbital tablet weighs 65 mg, then 12 tablets would weigh _____ mg.

19. If a scored digoxin (Lanoxin) tablet contains 0.25 mg of the medication, then one half of the tablet will contain

_____ mg of digoxin.

20. If a patient received three different intravenous drugs, each mixed in 50 ml of fluid over an 8-hour period, and also received 700 ml of prescribed intravenous fluid in that period, the total intravenous intake for the 8 hours would

be _____ ml.

Arabic numbers and Roman numerals
To review your competence in handling Roman numerals, solve the following problems. Then check your answers against those on page 40.

Write the following Arabic numbers as Roman numerals:

1. 17 _____
2. 54 _____
3. 490 _____
4. 82 _____
5. 7.5 _____
6. 15 _____
7. 75 _____
8. 110 _____
9. 21 _____
10. 204 _____

Write the following Roman numerals as Arabic numbers:

11. $\overline{\text{iv}}$ _____
12. XII _____
13. XVI _____
14. XXIX _____
15. MXL _____
16. XXXIV _____
17. CXL _____
18. XC _____

19. LXXV _____

20. $\bar{v}$ _____

21. $\overline{iss}$ _____

22. $\overline{\overline{iii}}$ _____

23. $\bar{x}$ _____

24. $\overline{viii}$ _____

25. XLVI _____

Apothecaries' conversions

To test your understanding of the apothecaries' system, answer the following questions. Check your answers against those on pages 40 and 41.

1. The volume of 1 drop of water equals _____ .

2. In a prescription, the abbreviation for 4½ drams is

_____ .

3. In a prescription, the abbreviation for 12 oz is

_____ .

4. In a prescription, the abbreviation for 2 drams is

_____ .

5. In a prescription, the abbreviation for 6 oz is

_____ .

6. ꝫ $\overline{iiss}$ = gr _____ .

7. ꝫ $\bar{i}$ = gr _____ .

8. M_x XVI ≈ gr _____ .

9. gr CCX = ꝫ _____ .

10. ꝫ $\overline{iv}$ = ꝫ _____ .

11. ꝫ XX = ꝫ _____ .

12. gr CCX = ꝫ _____ .

13. pt ¾ = ꝫ _____ .

14. qt $\overline{iiiss}$ = ꝫ _____ .

15. qt $\overline{ss}$ = ꝫ _____ .

16. gr CLXXX = ꝫ _____ .

17. gr CCC = ꝫ _____ .

18. ℥ iii = gr _____ .

19. gr XV = ℥ _____ .

20. ℥ ii = gr _____ .

21. M$_x$ x̄ = ℥ _____ .

22. 5 drops of water ≈ M$_x$ _____ .

23. M$_x$ XXX = ℥ _____ .

24. The weight of 1 drop of water equals _____ .

25. ℥ ¾ = M$_x$ _____ .

26. gr CXX = ℥ _____ .

27. 1 qt of antacid preparation contains _____ 1-dram doses.

28. A health care professional can pour _____ 4-oz bottles of a solution from a 1-gal stock bottle.

29. A 2-oz bottle of a tincture contains _____ 15-minim doses.

30. After 4 drams, 60 minims, and ¼ oz of paregoric are removed from a pint bottle, _____ drams are left.

31. How many ¼-grain doses of codeine can be prepared from a ½-oz stock bottle? _____

32. If 8 oz of cough expectorant contain 6 drams of ammonium chloride, 1 pt of the solution contains _____ drams of ammonium chloride.

Household conversions
Use these problems involving household system measurements to assess your progress. Check your answers against those on pages 41 and 42.

1. The abbreviation for drop is _____ .

2. 1 tsp = _____ gtt.

3. 3 Tbs = _____ tsp.

4. ½ cup = _____ Tbs.

5. 1 pt = _____ Tbs.

6. ½ tsp = _____ gtt.

7. 6 Tbs = _____ oz.

8. 1 pt and 8 oz = _____ cups.

9. 1 Tbs = _____ gtt.

10. 10 gtt = _____ tsp.

Equivalent measures among systems

These questions test your understanding of equivalent measures among systems. Answers follow on page 42.

1. A child is to receive 1 dram of cough medicine. This is the same as _____ tsp.

2. A physician's order reads *1 pt magnesium citrate.* This is equivalent to _____ oz.

3. A patient is to have an enema prepared with 1 L of water. At home, _____ qt of water may be used.

4. A child has been receiving 4 ml of a medication. At home, a measuring device labeled in teaspoons is to be used. The child should receive _____ tsp.

5. A physician's order reads *2 Tbs milk of magnesia.* This is equivalent to _____ ml.

ANSWERS TO PRACTICE PROBLEMS

Metric terms and conversions

1. metric
2. gram, milliliter, centimeter, and liter
3. meter
4. weight
5. liter
6. G (or GM)
7. L
8. mcg
9. ml
10. cc
11. $\frac{1}{1,000}$
12. 3, left
13. 3, right

14. 9
15. 1,800 ml = 1.8 L
16. 4,250 ml = 4.25 L
17. 374 mcl = 0.374 ml
18. 350 ml = 0.35 L
19. 10 cc = 10 ml
20. 1 L = 1,000 ml
21. 1 ml = 0.001 L
22. 58.5 L = 58,500 ml
23. 150 cc = 150 ml
24. 220 cc = 0.22 L
25. 57,820 cc = 57.82 L
26. 0.3 L = 300 ml
27. 1 L = 10 dl
28. 95 ml = 95 cc
29. 1 kg = 1,000 G
30. 1 G = 1,000,000 mcg
31. 1 G = 1,000 mg
32. 52 G = 0.052 kg
33. 6.2 G = 0.0062 kg
34. 732 G = 0.732 kg
35. 17 G = 17,000 mg
36. 0.17 G = 170 mg
37. 0.47 G = 470 mg
38. 286 G = 286,000 mg
39. 160 mcg = 0.16 mg
40. 1,970 mcg = 1.97 mg
41. 119,200 mcg = 119.2 mg
42. 600 mg = 0.6 G
43. 50,000 mcg = 0.05 G
44. 125 mcg = 0.125 mg
45. 3,270 mcg = 3.27 mg
46. 481,000 mcg = 0.481 G
47. 305 G = 0.305 kg

48. 1 mg = 1,000 mcg

49. 1 mg = 1,000,000 ng

50. 0.08 mcg = 80 ng

51. 5.5 G = 5,500 mg

52. 1 G = 1,000,000,000 ng

53. 33 kg = 33,000 G

54. 520 mg = 0.52 G

55. 0.732 G = 732,000 mcg

56. 0.47 G = 470 mg

57. 25 mcg = 0.025 mg

58. 0.083 mg = 83 mcg

59. 300 ng = 0.0003 mg

60. 50 mg = 50,000 mcg

Metric mathematics

1. 825.760 = 825.76 G

2. 3,225 ml

3. 1850.420 = 1,850.42 mg

4. 1.700 = 1.7 G

5. 2,487,245 mg

6. 650 ml

7. 4,044.344 G

8. 24,856 mcg

9. 30,369 mg

10. 1.51 G

11. 149 mg or 150 mg

12. 1.1455 = 1.146 G

13. 3 L

14. 335 ml

15. 400 mg

16. 55 mg

17. 750 mg

18. 780 mg

19. 0.125 mg

20. 850 ml

Arabic numbers and Roman numerals

1. 17 = XVII
2. 54 = LIV
3. 490 = CDXC
4. 82 = LXXXII
5. 7.5 = $\overline{\text{viiss}}$
6. 15 = XV
7. 75 = LXXV
8. 110 = CX
9. 21 = XXI
10. 204 = CCIV
11. $\overline{\text{iv}}$ = 4
12. XII = 12
13. XVI = 16
14. XXIX = 29
15. MXL = 1,040
16. XXXIV = 34
17. CXL = 140
18. XC = 90
19. LXXV = 75
20. $\overline{\text{v}}$ = 5
21. $\overline{\text{iss}}$ = 1½
22. $\overline{\text{iii}}$ = 3
23. $\overline{\text{x}}$ = 10
24. $\overline{\text{viii}}$ = 8
25. XLVI = 46

Apothecaries' conversions

1. M$_x$ $\overline{\text{i}}$
2. 4½ drams = ʒ $\overline{\text{ivss}}$
3. 12 oz = ʒ XII
4. 2 drams = ʒ $\overline{\text{ii}}$
5. 6 oz = ʒ $\overline{\text{vi}}$

6. ʒ $\overline{\text{iiss}}$ = gr CL

7. ʒ $\overline{\text{i}}$ = gr LX

8. M$_x$ XVI ≈ gr XVI

9. gr CCX = ʒ $\overline{\text{iiiss}}$

10. ʒ $\overline{\text{iv}}$ = ʒ XXXII

11. ʒ XX = ʒ $\overline{\text{iiss}}$

12. gr CCXL = ʒ $\overline{\text{iv}}$

13. pt ¾ = ʒ XII

14. qt $\overline{\text{iiiss}}$ = ʒ CXII

15. qt $\overline{\text{ss}}$ = ʒ CXXVIII

16. gr CLXXX = ʒ $\overline{\text{iii}}$

17. gr CCC = ʒ $\overline{\text{v}}$

18. ʒ $\overline{\text{iii}}$ = gr MCDXL

19. gr XV = ʒ ¼

20. ʒ $\overline{\text{ii}}$ = gr CXX

21. M$_x$ $\overline{\text{x}}$ = ʒ ⅙

22. 5 drops water ≈ M$_x$ $\overline{\text{v}}$

23. M$_x$ XXX = ʒ $\overline{\text{ss}}$

24. 1 drop of water weighs ≈ gr $\overline{\text{i}}$ wheat

25. ʒ ¾ = M$_x$ CCCLX

26. gr CXX = ʒ $\overline{\text{ii}}$

27. 1 qt of antacid = 256 1-dram doses

28. 1 gal solution = 32 4-oz bottles

29. 2-oz bottles of tincture = 64 15-M$_x$ doses

30. 1 pt (ʒ 128) − ʒ $\overline{\text{iv}}$, M$_x$ 60 (ʒ $\overline{\text{i}}$), + ¼ (ʒ $\overline{\text{ii}}$) = ʒ 121

31. ʒ $\overline{\text{ss}}$ = 960 gr ¼ doses

32. 12 (ʒ XII)

Household conversions

1. abbreviation for drop is gtt

2. 1 tsp = 60 gtt

3. 3 Tbs = 9 tsp

4. ½ cup = 8 Tbs

5. 1 pt = 32 Tbs
6. ½ tsp = 30 gtt
7. 6 Tbs = 3 oz
8. 1 pt, 8 oz = 3 cups
9. 1 Tbs = 180 gtt
10. 10 gtts = ⅙ tsp

Equivalent measures among systems

1. 1 tsp
2. 16 oz
3. 1 qt
4. 1 tsp
5. 30 ml

3

THE ADMINISTRATION PROCESS

In the first step of any drug distribution system, the physician must write a drug order, or prescription, for a patient. Because the order must pass through many steps in the system, a medication error can occur at any step and may produce severe consequences for the patient. You can prevent many medication errors by understanding and correctly using pharmacologic terminology. This chapter will help you do so by explaining how to read drug labels, interpret drug orders, and maintain records for all medications dispensed.

One way that institutions can help reduce medication errors is by using the unit-dose system of drug distribution. In this system, medications are contained in — and administered from — single-dose packages. They are dispensed in ready-to-use form whenever possible. For most medications, the pharmacy provides the patient care area no more than a 24-hour supply of doses at a time and maintains a profile for each patient.

Institutions that do not use the unit-dose system must rely on the individual prescription system in which transcription for the medication is sent to the pharmacy. The pharmacist fills the prescription using a container labeled for the patient. The drug is administered directly from the container. An error is less likely to be committed with this system than with the floor stock system because the drug supply is designated for only one patient. Implementation, however, is slow in the individual prescription system.

The oldest and least used system today, the floor stock system, maintains a stock supply of medications in the patient care area. With this system, you must be able to give the right drug dose in the correct dosage form from the available strengths in stock.

THE FIVE "RIGHTS" OF SAFE MEDICATION ADMINISTRATION

To avoid medication errors and ensure patient safety, be sure to check these five "rights" before administering any drug:
- the right drug
- the right dose
- the right route
- the right time
- the right patient.

With all systems, you must read and understand the drug order and the label of every drug dose dispensed.

Classic safeguards, known as the five "rights" of medication administration, help ensure patient safety when administering medications. (See *The five "rights" of safe medication administration.*)

READING IDENTIFICATION LABELS

Remember these three words before administering every dose of medication: *Read the label.* Always know what drug you are to give, how much to administer, and why. Label reading has become increasingly important as the institutional use of generic drugs has grown. The generic name is the accepted nonproprietary drug name, simplified from the chemical name. Many drug manufacturers use identical packaging for all generic drugs in the same dosage form. In many cases, the labels and containers for two different concentrations of the same drug may look alike except for the listing of the drug's concentration. *Reading drug labels* provides examples of look-alike labels that must be read carefully to avoid medication errors.

Safe drug administration requires comparing the physician's order, as transcribed on the patient's medication administration record (MAR), *directly* against the drug label *three times* before you administer the drug. The following example illustrates this procedure.

The patient's MAR indicates that the patient is to receive propranolol hydrochloride (Inderal) 10 mg P.O. as part of his 10 a.m. medications. Open the patient's medication drawer, find the drug labeled propranolol hydrochloride (Inderal) 10 mg, and note that it is in oral tablet form. Then, place the labeled drug *directly*

(Text continues on page 49.)

READING DRUG LABELS

The following five pairs of labels illustrate look-alikes that must be read carefully to avoid medication errors:

GUAIFENESIN SYRUP

These two containers are the same size, but the top container has a 5-ml dose of 100 mg, while the bottom one has a dose that is double this volume (10 ml) and contains 200 mg.

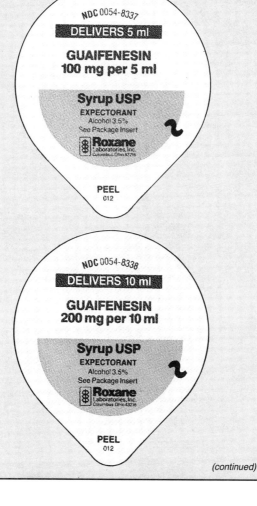

(continued)

READING DRUG LABELS *(continued)*

MORPHINE SULFATE ORAL SOLUTION
These two containers are the same size and they both hold morphine sulfate in a 10 mg/5 ml concentration. Yet the one on the top contains 5 ml and the one on the bottom contains 10 ml.

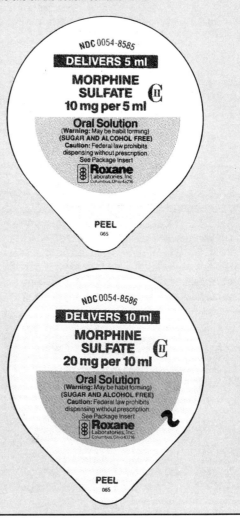

READING DRUG LABELS *(continued)*

THORAZINE

Although both of these bottles hold 4 oz of thorazine in a solution, they differ in one major way. The drug concentration in the bottle on the top is 10 mg/5 ml (2 mg/1 ml); the concentration in the bottle on the bottom is 30 mg/1 ml – 15 times greater than the other bottle. If these bottles were accidentally interchanged, serious consequences could result.

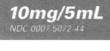

10mg/5mL
NDC 0007-5072-44

THORAZINE®
CHLORPROMAZINE HCl SYRUP

4 fl oz (118 mL)

SB SmithKline Beecham

1mL=30mg
NDC 0007-5047-44

THORAZINE®
CHLORPROMAZINE HCl CONCENTRATE

Intended for Institutional Use

4 fl oz (118 mL)

SB SmithKline Beecham

(continued)

READING DRUG LABELS *(continued)*

VERSED INJECTION

Each of these vials of Versed contains 5 ml. However, the vial at the top contains 1 mg/ml and the vial at the bottom contains 5 mg/ml—five times as much drug per milliliter as the first vial.

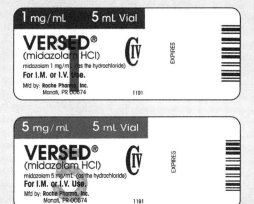

QUINIDINE SULFATE AND QUININE SULFATE

Although quinidine sulfate and quinine sulfate are similar-sounding drugs, they are not interchangeable. Quinidine sulfate is used to control arrhythmias; quinine sulfate is used to treat malaria.

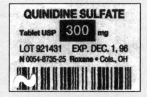

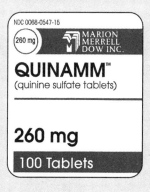

next to the transcribed order on the MAR, and carefully compare each part of the label and the order: propranolol hydrochloride, Inderal, and 10 mg.

If the drug is supplied in bulk or in a stock bottle, transfer one tablet from the supply to a medication container, pouring from the supply to the lid and then into the container without handling the tablet. Before returning the supply to the drawer or shelf, once again compare the label to the order on the MAR and again note whether this is the right time for administration. Remember, once a drug is removed from its container, you no longer can be certain that it is the correct drug—unless you've carefully compared the label to the MAR when pouring. When you get to the bedside, positively identify the patient, administer the now-unlabeled drug, and record the administration. (See *Comparing a drug order with a drug label,* pages 50 and 51.)

If the drug is supplied in a unit dose packet, do *not* remove it from the packet until you are at the patient's bedside and ready to administer it. At that time, after positively identifying the patient, make the third drug check, again by comparing the label directly to the order before removing it from the packet. Again, be sure to note whether this is the correct time to administer this drug. If so, administer the drug, and use the packet label for comparison when recording the administration.

READING DRUG ORDERS

As a nurse, you must be able to interpret the abbreviations that physicians use when they write medication prescriptions for patients (see *Common pharmacologic abbreviations,* pages 52 and 53).

These three guidelines will help you interpret drug orders:

■ The generic name of a drug should appear in lowercase letters only.

■ The trade, or brand, name of a drug should begin with a capital letter.

■ Drug abbreviations should be avoided, but when used should appear in all capital letters.

Review *Interpreting drug orders,* pages 54 and 55, for examples of drug orders and their interpretations.

Dealing with unclear drug orders

Once you know how to read drug orders, you will need to learn how to handle unclear orders. For example, many physicians

COMPARING A DRUG ORDER WITH A DRUG LABEL

Before administering a drug, carefully compare each part of the order on the medication administration record (MAR) with the drug label, holding the label next to the MAR to ensure accuracy. The following example illustrates the required steps:

1. Read the drug's generic name on the MAR (digoxin), and compare it to the drug's generic name on the label (digoxin).

2. Read the trade (proprietary) name on the MAR, if present (Lanoxin), and compare it to the proprietary name on the label (Lanoxin).

3. Read the dosage specified on the MAR (0.25 mg) and compare it to the dosage on the label (0.25 mg).

4. Read the route specified on the MAR (P.O.), and note the dosage form on the label (oral tablet).

5. Finally, note any special considerations on the MAR. (**Hold dose if apical rate is < 56/min and notify house officer.)

MEDICATION ADMINISTRATION RECORD

DATE ORD.	STOP DATE	MEDICATION DOSE	ROUTE FREQUENCY	R.N. INT.	HR.	8/8	8/9	9/10	9/11	8/12	8/13
8/8	8/11	digoxin (Lanoxin)		RU	10 A	X				X	D/C
		0.25 mg P.O. T.I.D. X			2 P	LB				X	P
		11 doses			6 P	QR AP-50				X	8/11
		**HOLD DOSE IF APICAL									
		RATE < 56/min AND									
		NOTIFY HOUSE OFFICER									

DRUG LABEL

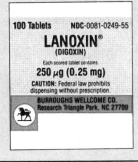

COMPARING A DRUG ORDER WITH A DRUG LABEL (continued)

As a further safeguard, be sure to compare the MAR and drug label *three times* before actually administering the drug: once when obtaining the drug from floor stock or the patient's supply, a second time before placing the drug in the medication cup or other administration device, and a third time before either replacing the stock drug bottle on the shelf or removing the drug from the unit dose packet at the patient's bedside.

Any discrepancies between the MAR and the drug label require your careful consideration. For instance, using the above example, suppose the MAR specified digoxin and the patient's drug packet was labeled only as Lanoxin; you would need to know that Lanoxin is the proprietary name for the drug digoxin. Suppose the drug packet was labeled digitoxin; you would need to recognize that this is a different digitalis glycoside that cannot be substituted for digoxin. Suppose the generic names were identical, but the packet contained an 0.125-mg tablet; you would have to know to administer two tablets to achieve the required dosage. Remember, only through scrupulous attention to such details can you ensure safe, error-free drug administration.

develop their own abbreviations and notations for drug orders; others have illegible handwriting. (See *Coping with difficult drug orders,* page 56, for samples.) In either case, the nurse must contact the physician for clarification. Remember, you are responsible for ensuring that the proper drug, strength, and dosage form are transcribed onto the Kardex or MAR, and given to the patient.

You will also need to know how to handle orders for drug doses in strengths that are not commercially available. For example, phenytoin is available only in 100-mg capsules or vials. If the physician orders phenytoin 300 mg P.O. or I.V., you will need to calculate the number of capsules or vials required to provide the correct dose. (Subsequent chapters provide detailed information about dosage calculation methods.)

In an outpatient setting, a physician or other individual licensed to prescribe medications may write a drug order on a prescription form and give it directly to the patient. In turn, the patient gives the order to a pharmacist, who dispenses the drug to the patient for home use. In a hospital, the prescriber writes the drug order on the physician's order sheet in the patient's

(Text continues on page 55.)

COMMON PHARMACOLOGIC ABBREVIATIONS

To transcribe medication orders and document drug administration accurately, review the following commonly used abbreviations for drug measurements, dosage forms, routes and times of administration, and related terms. Remember that abbreviations often are subject to misinterpretation, especially if written carelessly or quickly. If an abbreviation seems unusual or does not make sense to you, given your knowledge of the patient or the drug, *always* question the order, clarify the terms, and clearly *write out* the correct term in your revision and transcription.

DRUG AND SOLUTION MEASUREMENTS

cc	cubic centimeter	mEq	milliequivalent
ℨ	dram	mg	milligram
ℨ or oz	ounce	ml	milliliter
G or GM	gram	M_x	minim
gal	gallon	pt	pint
gr	grain	qt	quart
gtt	drop	ss̄	one half
kg	kilogram	Tbs	tablespoon
L	liter	tsp	teaspoon
mcg	microgram	U	unit

DRUG DOSAGE FORMS

cap	capsule	sp	spirits
DS	double strength	supp	suppository
elix	elixir	susp	suspension
LA	long-acting	syr	syrup
liq	liquid	tab	tablet
S.A.	sustained action	tinct or tr	tincture
S.R.	sustained release	ung or oint	ointment
sol	solution		

ROUTES OF DRUG ADMINISTRATION

A.D.	right ear	O.S.	left eye
A.S.	left ear	O.D.	right eye
A.U.	each ear	O.U.	each eye
I.M.	intramuscular	P.O. or p.o.	by mouth

COMMON PHARMACOLOGIC ABBREVIATIONS *(continued)*

ROUTES OF DRUG ADMINISTRATION *(continued)*

I.T.	intrathecal	R or P.R.	by rectum
I.V.	intravenous	ⓡ	right
IVPB	intravenous piggyback	ⓛ	left
		S.C. or SQ	subcutaneous
NGT	nasogastric tube	SL or sl	sublingual
V or P.V.	vaginally	S&S	swish and swallow

TIMES OF DRUG ADMINISTRATION

a.c.	before meals	q.h.	every hour
ad lib	as desired	q2h, q3h, etc.	every 2 hours, every 3 hours, etc.
b.i.d.	twice a day	q.i.d.	four times a day
h.s.	at bedtime	q.n.	every night
p.c.	after meals	q.o.d.	every other day
p.r.n.	as needed	STAT	immediately
q.a.m. or Q.M.	every morning	t.i.d.	three times a day
q.d. or Q.D.	every day		

MISCELLANEOUS ABBREVIATIONS

AMA	against medical advice	Rx	treatment, prescription
ASAP	as soon as possible	$\bar{s}$	without
$\bar{c}$	with	TO	telephone order
D/C or dc	discontinue	VO	verbal order
HO	house officer	≈	approximately equal to
KVO	keep vein open	>	greater than
MR	may repeat	<	less than
NKA	no known allergies	↑	increase
N.P.O.	nothing by mouth	↓	decrease

INTERPRETING DRUG ORDERS

The following examples illustrate how to read and interpret a wide range of drug orders.

DRUG ORDER	INTERPRETATION
Colace 100 mg P.O. b.i.d. p.c.	Give 100 mg of Colace by mouth twice a day after meals.
Vistaril 25 mg I.M. q3h p.r.n.	Give 25 mg of Vistaril intramuscularly every 3 hours, as needed.
↑ Duramorph to 6 mg I.V. q8h	Increase Duramorph to 6 mg intravenously every 8 hours.
folic acid 1 mg P.O. daily	Give 1 mg of folic acid by mouth daily.
Minipress 4 mg P.O. q6h, hold for sys BP < 120	Give 4 mg of Minipress by mouth every 6 hours; withhold drug if the systolic blood pressure falls below 120 mm Hg.
nifedipine 30 mg SL q4h	Give 30 mg of nifedipine sublingually every 4 hours.
Begin ASA 325 mg P.O. daily	Begin giving 325 mg of aspirin by mouth daily.
Begin Dyazide 1 cap P.O. q.a.m.	Begin giving 1 capsule of Dyazide by mouth every morning.
phenytoin 300 mg I.V. STAT	Give 300 mg of phenytoin intravenously immediately.
digoxin 0.25 mg P.O. daily	Give 0.25 mg of digoxin by mouth daily.
Zyloprim 100 mg P.O. b.i.d.	Give 100 mg of Zyloprim by mouth twice a day.
Benadryl 25-50 mg P.O. h.s. p.r.n. insomnia	Give 25 to 50 mg of Benadryl by mouth at bedtime, as needed, for insomnia.
Alupent inhaler 2 puffs q6h	Give 2 inhalations of Alupent every 6 hours.

INTERPRETING DRUG ORDERS (continued)

DRUG ORDER	INTERPRETATION
Nitrostat 1½ in q.i.d. to chest	Apply 1½ inches of Nitrostat ointment to chest four times a day.
Persantine 75 mg P.O. t.i.d.	Give 75 mg of Persantine by mouth three times a day.
aspirin gr $\bar{v}$ P.O. t.i.d.	Give 5 grains of aspirin by mouth three times a day.
Vasotec 2.5 mg P.O. daily	Give 2.5 mg of Vasotec by mouth daily.
1,000 ml D_5W I.V. $\bar{c}$ KCl 20 mEq at 100 ml/hr	Give 1,000 ml of dextrose 5% in water with 20 mEq of potassium chloride intravenously at a rate of 100 ml/hr.
D/C PCN I.V., start PCN-G 800,000 U P.O. q6h	Discontinue I.V. penicillin; start 800,000 units of penicillin G by mouth every 6 hours.
diphenhydramine 25-50 mg P.O. h.s. p.r.n.	Give 25 to 50 mg of diphenhydramine by mouth at bedtime, as needed.

chart. Because this order sheet must include complete patient information, it is usually stamped with the patient's admission data plate. Each order also must include all of the following information:

- date and time of the order
- name of drug (generic or proprietary)
- dosage form (in metric, apothecaries', or household measurements)
- route of administration (P.O., I.M., S.C., I.V., P.R., P.V., S.L., or topical; in some agencies, if the route is not given, the oral route may be assumed)
- administration schedule (as times per day or hour intervals)
- any restrictions or specifications related to the order
- the physician's signature (may follow a group of orders)
- the physician's issued registration number for controlled drugs (if applicable).

COPING WITH DIFFICULT DRUG ORDERS

The combination of poor handwriting and inappropriate abbreviations on a drug order can lead to confusion and medication errors. For any drug order that does not clearly state the drug name, amount, route of administration, and timing of administration, you should contact the physician. The examples below illustrate drug orders that need clarification.

Each physician has a unique handwriting style and possibly a unique way of writing medication orders. Thus, you bear a great responsibility to ensure that the proper drug, strength, and dosage form is ordered, transcribed onto the Kardex or medication administration record, and given to the patient.

Take note of the examples that follow.

FREEDOM HOSPITAL

DOCTOR'S ORDERS

INSTRUCTIONS

UNIT NO. 4 SOUTH , 432A
NAME   JOE JACKSON
ADDRESS 33 SHORT STREET
CITY   HOPE, NJ BIRTH 2·21·24

1. Each time a physicians writes a medication order, detach top copy and send to pharmacy.
2. Rule off unused lines after last copy (Pink) has been sent to pharmacy.

DO NOT USE THIS SHEET UNLESS A NUMBER SHOWS.

1

DATE	TIME	ORDERS	DOCTOR'S SIGNATURE	NURSE'S SIGNATURE
2/14	12³⁰ᵖ	*[illegible] 25/250 ? po q·d*		
		Captin 1 mg po BID		
		Benadryl 25 mg PO HS		
		ROM [illegible] to all extremities —		
		Soft diet patient may choose		
		PO fn MD		J. Adams RN
4/29		*DC Clonit*		
		DC Veracops		
		Kefzol 1.0 g IV q 6 h		
		V Sertaqui [illegible] 60 mg ℗ q 8 hrs		
6/30		*V Sertaqui [illegible] 60 mg ℗ q 12 h*		

Discharge diagnoses in order of decreasing priority must be supplied at time of patient's discharge.

If any of this required information is missing, you must question and clarify the order before signing the transcription. A contact copy or carbon copy of the order is sent to the pharmacy, where the drug is dispensed according to institutional policy. To limit the risk of error, make sure that only approved abbreviations are used in the order. The actual times at which the drug is administered depend on institutional policy (for drugs given a specific number of times per day) and on the drug's nature and onset and duration of action. These actual times are recorded on the MAR; the drug should be administered within $\frac{1}{2}$ hour either before or after the times specified.

MAINTAINING MEDICATION RECORDS

After the physician writes a drug order, you must verify the order by reviewing the drug, its therapeutic content, the dose (which may require checking the calculations), and the dosage form ordered. If a problem is detected, you should contact the physician before the drug order goes to the pharmacy. If the problem is not detected until after the drug order has gone to the pharmacy, you must contact the physician and the pharmacy.

Once the prescription has been verified, transcribe the order onto the medication charting form used in the institution. Drug order transcription requires close attention because a small error in rewriting an order can cause a major medication error. For medication charting, some institutions use a Kardex, a set of large index cards in a hinged file usually kept in the medication room or on the medication cart. Others use an MAR, an $8\frac{1}{2}$ in × 11 in chart form. Still others use a combination of both. And an increasing number of institutions enter medication charting information into a computer, which automatically generates a list of administration times for all scheduled medication doses. Use of computers should help decrease the incidence of drug errors caused by misinterpretation of handwriting.

No matter which type of medication charting form or system an institution uses, you should record certain standard information. (See *Sample medication record,* page 59, for an example.) This information is required so that medication records can serve as legal documents, if necessary, to prove that a drug dose was given. All of this information must appear legibly in ink on the Kardex or MAR. (See *Checking for errors in transcription*, page 60.)

Patient information

Record all patient information on the Kardex or MAR exactly as it appears on the patient's identification bracelet, stamping the Kardex or MAR with an addressograph plate, if possible. If this is not available, write the patient's full name, hospital identification number, unit number, and bed assignment on the Kardex or MAR. Also include all known allergies, even those that aren't drug related. If the patient has no known allergies, document this with the abbreviation NKA.

Dates

Certain dates must always appear on the Kardex or MAR: the date the prescription was written, the date the medication should begin (if different from the original order date), and the date the medication should be discontinued. In some institutions, the time the order is to be initiated is recorded with the date. This serves as a reference for the time to discontinue a drug when a limited time period is indicated.

Drug information

As part of the medication charting information, you should include the drug name, strength, dosage form, and route of administration.

Drug name
Always record the drug's full, preferably generic, name. If the physician ordered the drug using a particular proprietary name, record this name as well. Avoid using abbreviations, chemical symbols, research names, and special institutional names, which could cause medication errors or delays in therapy.

Drug strength
Be sure to document the actual amount of drug to be administered.

Drug dosage form
Indicate the dosage form as ordered by the physician. When recording the drug dosage form, consider the patient's special needs and the drug's physical form. For example, suppose a patient with a nasogastric tube needs medication for chronic

SAMPLE MEDICATION RECORD

The medication Kardex below illustrates the kind of information required on all types of medication administration forms. Although different institutions may use different forms, the information required is basically the same: patient information, date, drug information, time for and of administration, and your initials after you administer the drug.

INITIAL	SIGNATURE	INITIAL	SIGNATURE							

ALLERGIES

R = REFUSED O = OMITTED F = FASTING

ROUTINE MEDICATIONS

DATE ORD.	STOP DATE	MEDICATION DOSE	ROUTE FREQUENCY	R.N. INT.	HR.				DATE				

FREEDOM HOSPITAL

DIAGNOSIS & SURGERY · AGE · SEX · PHYSICIAN · ROOM · NAME

CHECKING FOR ERRORS IN TRANSCRIPTION

Drug administration errors often result from errors made in transcribing an order from the order sheet to the medication administration record (MAR) or medication Kardex. To avoid such errors, follow these guidelines:

■ Transcribe all orders in a quiet, distraction-free area, if possible.
■ Before signing the order sheet and initialing the MAR, carefully review all parts of the order.
■ Follow your institution's policy for reviewing orders. Some institutions require that all charts be reviewed for new orders each shift and that any orders written within 24 hours be checked. Others designate one shift (often the night shift) as responsible for reviewing all orders written in the preceding 24-hour period.

obstructive pulmonary disease, and the physician orders sustained-action theophylline. Because of the patient's special needs, the tablets would have to be crushed to be administered. But because of the drug's physical form, sustained-action tablets, crushing would destroy its integrity and possibly its therapeutic action. In such a case, you would have to contact the physician to discuss and resolve the problem.

Route of administration
Always specify the route of administration. This is especially important for drugs that may be given by two different routes; for example, orally or rectally, as with acetaminophen (Tylenol). Some parenteral medications can be given by only one correct route; for example, NPH insulin may be given subcutaneously but not intravenously.

Time of administration

The physician's order includes a desired administration schedule, such as t.i.d. or q6h. This is transcribed on the MAR and then converted into actual times based on the institution's scheduled times (t.i.d. may be 9-1-5 in one institution and 10-2-6 in another), the availability and characteristics of the drug, or the drug's onset and duration of action (b.i.d. may be 10 and 6 or 10 and 10; q6h may be 10-4-10-4 or 12-6-12-6).

Some institutions have separate MARs or specially designated areas of the MAR for recording single drug orders or special drug orders (for example, drugs given as needed). Other institutions include these drugs on the daily MAR; in the latter case, one must carefully distinguish these drugs from scheduled medications.

Initials

Usually, the person who transcribes the order to the MAR from the order sheet indicates this by signing the order sheet and initialing the order on the MAR. If someone other than a nurse transcribes the order, you must co-sign the order sheet and the MAR.

Before administering medications, you should read the physician's orders to ensure that the MAR accurately reflects the orders, including any recent orders or changes in orders. Many institutions require you to initial the physician's order sheet, on the line following the last order, to indicate that all orders have been transcribed correctly onto the MAR.

Documenting on the medication record

After administering a drug, add the following information to the MAR.

Dosage

If the dosage you administer varies in any way from the dosage strength or amount ordered, note this fact in a special area on the MAR or in the patient's progress notes. For example, you would document whether the patient refused to take a medication, consumed only part of the medication, or vomited shortly after ingesting the medication.

Route of administration

When administering a drug by a parenteral route, record the injection site to facilitate site rotation. Most MAR forms include a numbered list of recognized sites so that you can record the site by its number in the limited space available. If you administer a drug by a different route than that originally specified, you must so indicate, along with the reason and authorization for the change.

Time of administration

Immediately after administering a drug, accurately document the time of administration to help prevent repeat administration of the same drug dose. For scheduled drugs (those with a planned time schedule), you will usually do so by initialing the appropriate time slot for the date you are giving the drug. Scheduled drug administration is considered on time if given within ½ hour before or after the ordered time. For unscheduled drugs (single doses, STATs, and p.r.n.s), indicate the exact time of administration in the appropriate time slot. If a drug is not given as scheduled, be sure to document the reason for the delay or omission. Some MARs have a place for this information; in others, you will record the information in the patient's progress notes. Institutional policy may require you to initial and circle the particular time frame missed on the MAR to draw attention to the omission of the dose.

Identifying initials

When you administer a drug, verify that the dose was given by initialing the MAR in the appropriate time slot. Make sure your initials are clearly legible and different from those of other nurses on the unit who might give drugs to this patient. (Use your middle initial for clarification if necessary.) Then, identify the initials as yours by recording them in the signature section of the MAR, along with your signature and title. Your signature and initial identification must appear on every record that you have initialed when administering drugs. Always sign your initials in the same way on every record.

Handling omitted medication doses

Facility policies vary greatly regarding documentation of medications that are not administered when scheduled. In any facility, however, you must record that the medication was not given and must provide a reason for the omission in the nurse's notes or MAR. (Some common reasons include patient refusal to take the medication, NPO status, or inadequate apical pulse or blood pressure for cardiovascular drug administration.) Also, you should always fill in the time slot on the MAR; leaving it blank suggests that a medication administration error was made and that the patient did not receive the prescribed medication.

Other medication records

Some institutions require you to document all drugs that a patient receives on a single Kardex or MAR. Other institutions use separate forms for p.r.n. drugs, large-volume parenterals, one-time-only doses, and treatment items (dermatologic and ophthalmic medications dispensed in bottles or tubes).

Federal and state laws regulate the dispensing, administration, and documentation of controlled substances. When a controlled

SAMPLE PERPETUAL INVENTORY RECORD

Federal and state laws require special documentation for administering controlled substances, usually on a form like this one:

FREEDOM HOSPITAL   000101
RECORD OF CONTROLLED SUBSTANCES DISPOSITION

DIVISION _____

COST CENTER # _____

PREPARED BY: _____

DELIVERED BY: _____

DATE _____

NURSE SIG. _____

AMOUNT DELIVERED _____

REMOVE THIS FORM AND RETURN TO PHARMACY AFTER NURSE'S SIGNATURE IS OBTAINED.

DATE	TIME	PATIENT'S FULL NAME	PHYSICIAN'S NAME	NURSE'S SIGNATURE	AMT GIVEN	AMT WASTED	WITNESS SIGNATURE	AMT REMAINING
	AM/PM							
	AM/PM							
	AM/PM							
	AM/PM							
	AM/PM							
	AM/PM							
	AM/PM							
	AM/PM							
	AM/PM							
	AM/PM							
	AM/PM							
	AM/PM							
	AM/PM							
	AM/PM							
	AM/PM							
	AM/PM							
	AM/PM							

HOW TO USE THIS FORM:
1. NUMBER ON THIS FORM MUST COINCIDE WITH NUMBER ON CONTAINER
2. ALL ENTRIES MUST BE IN INDELIBLE INK
3. DOSAGE WASTED, DISCARDED, OR LOST MUST HAVE SHORT EXPLANATION AND SIGNATURE OF SECOND PERSON (WITNESS SIGNATURE)

ABOVE RECORD VERIFIED AS COMPLETE (NURSING)
_____ DATE _____

ABOVE RECORD VERIFIED AS COMPLETE (PHARMACY)
_____ DATE _____

substance is issued to a patient care area, a perpetual inventory record like the one above is issued with it to document the disposition of each dose and to record the name of the nurse responsible for administering each dose.

If a physician orders a controlled substance for a patient, you must record its administration on the Kardex or MAR and on the perpetual inventory record. When the dose is removed from the double-locked storage site, record the following information on the perpetual inventory record: the date and time the dose is removed, the patient's full name, the physician's name, the drug's dose, and your signature. If any of the dose must be discarded, two nurses must verify the amount discarded and sign the form.

PRACTICE PROBLEMS

Translate the following physician's orders. To check your answers, see pages 70 to 73.

1. Compazine 10 mg I.M. q6h p.r.n. for N/V

_____

_____

2. acetaminophen supp 650 mg P.R. q4h p.r.n. for T > 102®

_____

_____

3. Nembutal 100 mg P.O. h.s. p.r.n.

_____

_____

4. digoxin 0.125 mg P.O. daily

_____

_____

5. Transderm-Nitro 10, 1 patch h.s.

_____

_____

6. lidocaine 50 mg I.V. bolus at 25 mg/minute STAT and q5minute × 1 p.r.n.

_____

_____

7. regular insulin 30 U I.V. stat

_____

_____

8. D/C lidocaine I.V. drip

_____

_____

9. Bronkometer inhaler 2 puffs q4h p.r.n.

_____

_____

10. Cefadyl 1 G I.M. q6h

11. nifedipine 10 mg SL q8h

12. Tenormin 50 mg P.O. daily

13. hydrochlorothiazide 25 mg P.O. daily

14. Demerol 50-75 mg I.M. q4h p.r.n. for pain

15. hydroxyzine 50 mg I.M. q4h p.r.n. for anxiety

16. $FeSO_4$ 325 mg P.O. t.i.d.

17. Tylenol gr $\overline{x}$ P.O. q6h p.r.n. for headache

18. Mylanta 30 ml P.O. q.i.d. 1h p.c. & h.s.

19. Dalmane 15 mg P.O. h.s. p.r.n. MR $\times$ 1

20. Change I.V. from D_5LR to LR

_____

_____

21. KCl 20 mEq P.O. q4h $\times$ 2 doses

_____

_____

22. hydrocortisone 50 mg P.O. b.i.d.

_____

_____

23. Dilantin 100 mg P.O. b.i.d.

_____

_____

24. Theo-Dur 200 mg P.O. q12h

_____

_____

25. Procardia 20 mg P.O. t.i.d.

_____

_____

26. oxacillin 1 G I.V.P.B. q6h $\times$ 2 doses

_____

_____

27. Dicloxacillin 500 mg P.O. q6h

_____

_____

28. $D_5\frac{1}{2}NS$ I.V. at 80 ml/h

_____

_____

29. heparin 5,000 Units S.C. q12h

_____

_____

30. gentamicin ophthalmic solution 0.3% 1 gtt O.D. q4h

_____

_____

31. milk of magnesia 2 Tbs P.O. h.s. p.r.n. for constipation

_____

_____

32. pseudoephedrine 30 mg P.O. q4-6h p.r.n. for congestion

_____

_____

33. ampicillin 2 G I.V.P.B. q4h

_____

_____

34. acetaminophen supp gr XX P.R. q4h p.r.n. for T > 102®

_____

_____

35. phenytoin susp 300 mg per NGT q.a.m. and 200 mg per NGT q.p.m.

_____

_____

36. 1,000 ml D_5W to KVO

_____

_____

37. amikacin 450 mg I.V.P.B. in 200 ml diluent over 60 m q12h

_____

_____

38. Change I.V. to 1,000 ml D_5W at 200 ml/h

_____

_____

39. 1,000 ml $D_5\frac{1}{2}NS$ I.V. $\bar{c}$ KCl 20 mEq at 125 ml/h

---

40. nafcillin 1 G I.V.P.B. in 50 ml NSS q6h $\times$ 4 doses, then 500 mg P.O. q6h $\times$ 10 days, then D/C

---

41. codeine gr $\overline{ss}$ P.O. q3h p.r.n. for pain

---

42. diazepam 5 mg I.M. q6h p.r.n. for muscle spasm

---

43. Anusol supp $\bar{i}$ PR p.r.n. for hemorrhoidal pain

---

44. Benadryl 25 mg P.O. STAT

---

45. ↓ D_5W I.V. to 200 ml/h

---

46. meperidine 50 mg P.O. q3-4h p.r.n. for pain

---

47. colchicine 0.6 mg P.O. b.i.d. $\bar{c}$ milk

---

48. ibuprofen 300 mg P.O. q.i.d.

---

49. D/C Valium

50. Ativan 2 mg P.O. t.i.d. and 4 mg h.s.

51. Dulcolax supp ī PR p.r.n. for constipation

52. TPN at 100 ml/h

53. simethicone 40 mg P.O. p.c. p.r.n.

54. quinidine sulfate 300 mg P.O. q6h

55. Metamucil 2 tsp in ℥ v̄iīi H₂O or juice P.O. daily p.r.n.

56. nystatin susp (100,000 U/ml) 5 ml q.i.d. S.&S.

57. guaifenesin ℥ īī q.i.d.

58. propranolol 40 mg b.i.d. a.c., hold if systolic BP < 100

59. ↓ clindamycin to 600 mg I.V. q6h

60. Aldomet 250 mg t.i.d. × 48h, then ↑ to 500 mg t.i.d.

ANSWERS TO PRACTICE PROBLEMS

1. Administer 10 mg of Compazine by intramuscular injection every 6 hours, as needed, for nausea or vomiting.

2. Administer a 650-mg acetaminophen suppository rectally every 4 hours, as needed, for temperature above 102° F (measured rectally).

3. Administer 100 mg of Nembutal by mouth at bedtime, as needed.

4. Administer 0.125 mg of digoxin by mouth daily.

5. Apply a 10-mg patch of Transderm-Nitro at bedtime.

6. Immediately administer 50 mg of lidocaine by intravenous bolus infusion over a 2-minute period (at an administration rate of 25 mg/minute); if necessary, repeat the dose after 5 minutes, one time only.

7. Immediately administer 30 units of regular insulin intravenously.

8. Discontinue the intravenous infusion of lidocaine.

9. Administer two oral inhalations of Bronkometer every 4 hours, as needed.

10. Administer 1 gram of Cefadyl by intramuscular injection every 6 hours.

11. Administer 10 mg of nifedipine sublingually every 8 hours.

12. Administer 50 mg of Tenormin by mouth every day.

13. Administer 25 mg of hydrochlorothiazide by mouth every day.

14. Administer 50 to 75 mg of Demerol by intramuscular injection every 4 hours, as needed, depending on the severity of pain.

15. Administer 50 mg of hydroxyzine hydrochloride by intramuscular injection every 4 hours, as needed, for anxiety.

16. Administer 325 mg of ferrous sulfate by mouth three times a day.

17. Administer 10 grains of Tylenol by mouth every 6 hours, as needed, for headache.

18. Administer 30 ml of Mylanta by mouth four times a day, 1 hour after each meal and at bedtime.

19. Administer 15 mg of Dalmane by mouth at bedtime, as needed. Repeat once during the night if necessary.

20. Change the patient's intravenous fluid from dextrose 5% in Ringer's lactate solution to plain Ringer's lactate solution.

21. Administer two 20-milliequivalent doses of potassium chloride by mouth, 4 hours apart.

22. Administer 50 mg of hydrocortisone by mouth twice a day.

23. Administer 100 mg of Dilantin by mouth twice a day.

24. Administer 200 mg of Theo-Dur by mouth every 12 hours.

25. Administer 20 mg of Procardia by mouth three times a day.

26. Administer two 1-gram doses of oxacillin by piggyback intravenous infusion, 6 hours apart.

27. Administer 500 mg of dicloxacillin sodium by mouth every 6 hours.

28. Administer 5% dextrose in 0.45% normal saline solution by intravenous infusion at a rate of 80 ml/hour.

29. Administer 5,000 units of heparin sodium by subcutaneous injection every 12 hours.

30. Place 1 drop of 0.3% gentamicin ophthalmic solution in the right eye every 4 hours.

31. Administer 2 tablespoons of milk of magnesia at bedtime, as needed, for constipation.

32. Administer 30 mg of pseudoephedrine hydrochloride by mouth every 4 to 6 hours, as needed, for congestion.

33. Administer 2 grams of ampicillin by piggyback intravenous infusion every 4 hours.

34. Administer a 20-grain acetaminophen suppository rectally every 4 hours, as needed, for temperature above 102° F (measured rectally).

35. Administer 300 mg of phenytoin suspension every morning and 200 mg every evening through a nasogastric tube.

36. Administer 1,000 ml of dextrose 5% in water by intravenous infusion at a rate designed to keep the vein patent (open).

37. Administer 450 mg of amikacin sulfate, mixed in 200 ml of the recommended diluent, by piggyback intravenous infusion over a 60-minute period every 12 hours.

38. Change the intravenous infusion to 1,000 ml of 5% dextrose in water delivered at a rate of 200 ml/hour.

39. Add 20 milliequivalents of potassium chloride to 1,000 ml of dextrose 5% in 0.45% normal saline solution, and administer by intravenous infusion at a rate of 125 ml/hour.

40. Administer 1 gram of nafcillin diluted in 50 ml of normal saline solution every 6 hours for four doses, then change to 500 mg by mouth every 6 hours for 10 days, then discontinue.

41. Administer ½ grain of codeine by mouth every 3 hours, as necessary, for pain.

42. Administer 5 mg of diazepam by intramuscular injection every 6 hours, as necessary, for muscle spasm.

43. Insert one Anusol suppository rectally, as needed, for hemorrhoidal pain.

44. Immediately administer 25 mg of Benadryl by mouth.

45. Decrease the intravenous infusion rate of dextrose 5% in water to 200 ml each hour.

46. Administer 50 mg of meperidine by mouth every 3 to 4 hours, as necessary, for pain.

47. Administer 0.6 mg of colchicine by mouth with milk twice a day.

48. Administer 300 mg of ibuprofen by mouth four times a day.

49. Discontinue Valium administration.

50. Administer 2 mg of Ativan by mouth three times a day, then administer 4 mg at bedtime.

51. Insert one Dulcolax suppository rectally, as necessary, for constipation.

52. Administer total parenteral nutrition as formulated at a rate of 100 ml/hour.

53. Administer 40 mg of simethicone by mouth after meals, as necessary.

54. Administer 300 mg of quinidine sulfate by mouth every 6 hours.

55. Administer 2 teaspoons of Metamucil mixed in 8 ounces of water or juice by mouth daily, as necessary.

56. Administer 5 ml of nystatin suspension (strength: 100,000 units/ml), have patient swish in mouth, then swallow.

57. Administer 2 drams of guaifenesin four times a day.

58. Administer 40 mg of propranolol twice a day before meals. Hold the dose if the patient's systolic blood pressure falls below 100 mm Hg.

59. Decrease clindamycin dosage to 600 mg administered intravenously every 6 hours.

60. Administer 250 mg of Aldomet three times a day for 48 hours (for a total of six doses); then increase the dosage to 500 mg three times a day.

CALCULATING ENTERAL DRUG DOSAGES

E nteral medications (drugs that are introduced into the body through the gastrointestinal [GI] tract) may be administered by mouth, feeding tube, or suppository. They must not be confused with parenteral medications (drugs that are introduced through a route other than the GI tract) and must *never* be administered by the parenteral route.

Whether an enteral drug comes in liquid, tablet, topical, or injectable form, it may require dilution, more precise measurement, reconstitution, breaking (of scored tablets), or some other alteration to provide an exact dose. If your facility does not use the unit-dose system of drug distribution, you'll need to calculate dosages and alter drugs, especially for pediatric and geriatric patients and for others who need carefully individualized doses. (See Chapter 7, Other Considerations.) This chapter applies the mathematical principles presented in Chapter 1, Review of Mathematics, to dosage calculations and solution preparation for enteral medications.

The inexact nature of conversions and computations

Converting drug measures from one system to another and then determining the amount of a dosage form to give often results in inexact dosages. A rounding error during computation or discrepancies in the dosage to give may occur, depending on the conversion factor used in the calculation. You may determine a precise amount of drug to be given, only to find that administering that amount is impossible. You may determine, for example, that a patient should receive 0.97 tablet. The following general rule avoids calculation errors and discrepancies between theoretical and real dosages: *No more than a 10% variation should exist between the dose ordered and the dose given.* Thus, if 0.97 tablet should be given, you could give 1 tablet.

You may encounter such discrepancies when converting doses of aspirin or acetaminophen from grains to milligrams. Depending on which conversion factor you use, gr $\bar{\text{i}}$ can equal 60 or 65 mg; thus, gr $\bar{\text{x}}$ can equal 600 or 650 mg. If the tablets were labeled as 325 mg each, you would give two tablets, even if your calculation showed 600 mg to be correct. Since 10% of 600 is 60, you could give up to 660 mg. Remember that if a large amount of drug (600 mg) is necessary to produce an effect, 50 or 60 mg more will not alter the effect significantly. On the other hand, if a small amount of drug (0.125 mg) is required to provide the desired effect, even a small increase could result in an overdose, depending on the drug's therapeutic range. In this case, following the 10% rule, you could give no more than 0.1375 mg.

RATIO AND FRACTION PROPORTION METHODS

Nurses frequently use the ratio and fraction proportion methods to calculate drug dosages and to convert between measurement systems.

Review of ratios and proportions

Because dosage calculations require your complete understanding of several mathematical concepts, this section reviews the basics of the ratio and fraction proportion methods, describes how you apply these methods to many types of dosage calculations, and provides step-by-step examples of these procedures.

Terms and functions

A *ratio* is a mathematical expression of the relationship between two different things. A *proportion* is a set of two equal ratios. A ratio may be expressed with a fraction, such as ⅓, or with a colon, such as 1:3. This text uses the term *ratio* when referring to those expressed with colons and *fraction* when referring to those written in fraction form.

When ratios are expressed as fractions in a proportion, their *cross products* are equal, as indicated below:

$$\frac{2}{4} \diagup\!\!\!\!\diagdown \frac{5}{10} \qquad 2 \times 10 = 4 \times 5$$

Proportion   *Cross products*

When ratios are expressed using colons in a proportion, the product of the means equals the product of the extremes:

Proportion   *Product of means and extremes*

means

3:30 :: 4:40 $30 \times 4 = 3 \times 40$

extremes

Whether fractions or ratios are used in a proportion, the units must appear in the same order on both sides of the equation. When the ratios are expressed as fractions, the units in the numerators must be the same and the units in the denominators must be the same (although they do not have to be the same as the units in the numerators). The example below demonstrates this principle:

$$\frac{\text{mg}}{\text{kg}} = \frac{\text{mg}}{\text{kg}}$$

If the ratios in a proportion are expressed with colons, the units of the first term on the left side of the double colon must be the same as the units in the first term on the right side. In other words, the units of the mean on one side of the double colon must match the units of the extreme on the other side, and vice versa. The example below demonstrates this principle:

mg:kg :: mg:kg

When you perform calculations, use ratios in colon or fractional form — whichever is more comfortable for you.

Tips for use
Several important tips will simplify dosage calculations with the ratio and fraction proportion methods.

Leave units of measure in the calculation. This tip will help protect you from one of the most common dosage calculation errors — the incorrect unit of measure. When you leave units of measure in the calculation, those in the numerator and the denominator cancel each other out and leave the correct unit of measure in the answer. The following example uses the units of measure in a calculation for a drug with a usual dose of 4 mg/kg for a 10-kg patient:

- State the problem in a proportion:

4 mg:1 kg :: X mg:10 kg

▪ Solve for X by applying the principle that the product of the means equals the product of the extremes:

$$1 \text{ kg} \times \text{X mg} = 4 \text{ mg} \times 10 \text{ kg}$$

▪ Divide and cancel out the units of measure that appear in the numerator and denominator:

$$X = \frac{4 \text{ mg} \times 10 \text{ k\cancel{g}}}{1 \text{ k\cancel{g}}}$$

$$X = 40 \text{ mg}$$

Watch the number of zeros and decimal places. An error in the number of zeros or decimal places in a calculation can cause a *tenfold* or greater dosage error. Suppose you receive an order to administer 0.1 mg of epinephrine S.C., but the only epinephrine on hand is a 1-ml ampule that contains 1 mg of epinephrine. To calculate the volume for injection, you may use the fraction proportion method.

▪ State the problem in a proportion:

$$\frac{\text{X ml}}{0.1 \text{ mg}} = \frac{1 \text{ ml}}{1 \text{ mg}}$$

▪ Solve for X by cross multiplying:

$$\text{X ml} \times 1 \text{ mg} = 0.1 \text{ mg} \times 1 \text{ ml}$$

▪ Divide and cancel out the units of measure that appear in the numerator and denominator, carefully checking the decimal placement:

$$X = \frac{0.1 \text{ m\cancel{g}} \times 1 \text{ ml}}{1 \text{ m\cancel{g}}}$$

$$X = 0.1 \text{ ml}$$

Recheck calculations that seem unusual. For example, if a calculation yields an answer that suggests you administer 25 tablets, 200 ml of an oral suspension, or a 20-ml I.M. injection, you probably have made a calculation error and should recheck your figures carefully. If you still have any doubt about your methods or results, review your calculations with another nurse.

Use a calculator. Hand-held calculators can improve the accuracy and speed of calculations. But remember: An electronic calculator cannot guarantee the accuracy of your dosage calculations. You must set up the proportions carefully and watch the units of measure and decimal places for the results to be reliable and accurate.

Converting between measurement systems

In clinical practice, you frequently see more than one system of measurement used in the same prescription. Before units such as grains and grams can be combined, however, you must convert all quantities to the same measurement system — metric, apothecaries', household, or avoirdupois.

When you convert a measurement from one system to another, you will obtain an *approximate* or practical equivalent, not an exact one. This is permissible because up to 10% variation between the dose ordered and the dose administered is considered acceptable in most cases. To convert, follow four basic steps:

1. Set up a ratio or fraction with the known conversion factor. Remember, when more than one conversion factor is available, use the one that fits your problem most easily. For example, gr i̇ can equal 60 mg, 64 mg, or 65 mg.

2. Set up a ratio or fraction with the unknown quantity and the quantity to be converted.

3. State these ratios or fractions in a proportion. Be sure that the units appear in the same order on both sides of the double colon or equal sign.

4. Solve for X, either by applying the principle that the product of the means equals the product of the extremes (when using the ratio method) or by cross multiplying (when using the fraction method).

Patient situations: Conversions between grains and milligrams

1. A physician orders ASA gr v̄ for a patient, but the aspirin tablets are available in milligrams only. How many milligrams should you administer?

By applying the four-step process, you can make the conversion and determine the correct dosage to give.

■ Set up the first ratio with the conversion factor:

1 gr:65 mg

■ Set up the second ratio with the unknown quantity in the appropriate position:

5 gr:X mg

■ Use these ratios in a proportion:

1 gr:65 mg :: 5 gr:X mg

■ Solve for X by applying the principle that the product of the means equals the product of the extremes:

$$65 \text{ mg} \times 5 \text{ gr} = 1 \text{ gr} \times X \text{ mg}$$

$$X = \frac{65 \text{ mg} \times 5 \text{ g\!\!\!/r}}{1 \text{ g\!\!\!/r}}$$

$$X = 325 \text{ mg}$$

2. Colchicine is available in 0.6-mg tablets. What is the equivalent in grains?

■ Set up a fraction with the conversion factor:

$$\frac{1 \text{ gr}}{65 \text{ mg}}$$

■ Set up a fraction with the unknown quantity:

$$\frac{X \text{ gr}}{0.6 \text{ mg}}$$

■ Use these fractions in a proportion:

$$\frac{X \text{ gr}}{0.6 \text{ mg}} = \frac{1 \text{ gr}}{65 \text{ mg}}$$

■ Solve for X by cross multiplying:

$$X \text{ gr} \times 65 \text{ mg} = 0.6 \text{ mg} \times 1 \text{ gr}$$

$$X = \frac{0.6 \text{ m\!\!\!/g} \times 1 \text{ gr}}{65 \text{ m\!\!\!/g}}$$

$$X = 0.009 \text{ gr}$$

If you had to convert 0.6 mg of colchicine to micrograms (mcg), you would follow the same steps.

■ Set up a fraction with the conversion factor:

$$\frac{1,000 \text{ mcg}}{1 \text{ mg}}$$

■ Set up a fraction with the unknown quantity:

$$\frac{X \text{ mcg}}{0.6 \text{ mg}}$$

■ Use these fractions in a proportion:

$$\frac{X \text{ mcg}}{0.6 \text{ mg}} = \frac{1,000 \text{ mcg}}{1 \text{ mg}}$$

- Solve for X by cross multiplying:

$$X \text{ mcg} \times 1 \text{ mg} = 0.6 \text{ mg} \times 1,000 \text{ mcg}$$

$$X = \frac{0.6 \text{ mg} \times 1,000 \text{ mcg}}{1 \text{ mg}}$$

$$X = 600 \text{ mcg}$$

Patient situations: Conversions between pounds and kilograms

1. A patient weighs 217 pounds, which you must convert to a metric weight to determine the correct dose to adminster.

To make conversions between pounds in the household system and kilograms in the metric system, you will need to use the conversion factor 1 kg = 2.2 lb in the four-step process:

- Set up the first ratio with the conversion factor:

$$1 \text{ kg}:2.2 \text{ lb}$$

- Set up the second ratio with the the unknown quantity:

$$X \text{ kg}: 217 \text{ lb}$$

- Use these ratios in a proportion:

$$1 \text{ kg}:2.2 \text{ lb} :: X \text{ kg}:217 \text{ lb}$$

- Solve for X by applying the principle that the product of the means equals the product of the extremes:

$$2.2 \text{ lb} \times X \text{ kg} = 1 \text{ kg} \times 217 \text{ lb}$$

$$X = \frac{1 \text{ kg} \times 217 \text{ lb}}{2.2 \text{ lb}}$$

$$X = 98.6 \text{ kg}$$

2. Suppose you need to determine how many pounds are in 70 kg, the average patient weight on which many adult drug dosages are based.

- Set up a fraction with the conversion factor:

$$\frac{2.2 \text{ lb}}{1 \text{ kg}}$$

- Set up a fraction with the unknown quantity:

$$\frac{X \text{ lb}}{70 \text{ kg}}$$

■ Use these fractions in a proportion, ensuring that the units appear in the same order on both sides of the equal sign:

$$\frac{X \text{ lb}}{70 \text{ kg}} = \frac{2.2 \text{ lb}}{1 \text{ kg}}$$

■ Solve for X by cross multiplying:

$$X \text{ lb} \times 1 \text{ kg} = 2.2 \text{ lb} \times 70 \text{ kg}$$

$$X = \frac{2.2 \text{ lb} \times 70 \text{ kg}}{1 \text{ kg}}$$

$$X = 154 \text{ lb}$$

Patient situations: Conversions between teaspoons and milliliters

1. A drug order calls for 2½ tsp of Bactrim suspension twice daily. You must convert this to the metric system. What is the equivalent in milliliters?

To convert between teaspoons in the household system and milliliters in the metric system, you must use the conversion factor 5 ml = 1 tsp in the four-step process:

■ Set up the first ratio with the conversion factor:

5 ml:1 tsp

■ Set up the second ratio with the unknown metric quantity:

X ml:2.5 tsp

■ Use these ratios in a proportion:

5 ml:1 tsp :: X ml:2.5 tsp

■ Solve for X by applying the principle that the product of the means equals the product of the extremes:

$$1 \text{ tsp} \times X \text{ ml} = 5 \text{ ml} \times 2.5 \text{ tsp}$$

$$X = \frac{5 \text{ ml} \times 2.5 \text{ tsp}}{1 \text{ tsp}}$$

$$X = 12.5 \text{ ml}$$

2. A child is given 7.5 ml of an antibiotic suspension three times daily. You must tell the parent how much antibiotic suspension to give the child at home. What is the equivalent in teaspoons?

■ Set up a fraction with the conversion factor:

$$\frac{1 \text{ tsp}}{5 \text{ ml}}$$

- Set up a fraction with the unknown household quantity:

$$\frac{\text{X tsp}}{7.5 \text{ ml}}$$

- Use these fractions in a proportion:

$$\frac{\text{X tsp}}{7.5 \text{ ml}} = \frac{1 \text{ tsp}}{5 \text{ ml}}$$

- Solve for X by cross multiplying:

$$\text{X tsp} \times 5 \text{ ml} = 1 \text{ tsp} \times 7.5 \text{ ml}$$

$$\text{X} = \frac{1 \text{ tsp} \times 7.5 \text{ ml}}{5 \text{ ml}}$$

$$\text{X} = 1.5 \text{ tsp}$$

Patient situations: Conversions among ounces, milliliters, and tablespoons

1. A drug order calls for milk of magnesia 1½ oz h.s. You must convert this to the metric system. What is the equivalent in milliliters?

To convert ounces to milliliters, you must use the conversion factor 1 oz = 30 ml in the four-step process:

- Set up the first ratio with the conversion factor:

$$1 \text{ oz:30 ml}$$

- Set up the second ratio with the unknown metric quantity:

$$1.5 \text{ oz:X ml}$$

- Use these ratios in a proportion:

$$1 \text{ oz:30 ml} :: 1.5 \text{ oz:X ml}$$

- Solve for X by applying the principle that the product of the means equals the product of the extremes:

$$30 \text{ ml} \times 1.5 \text{ oz} = 1 \text{ oz} \times \text{X ml}$$

$$\text{X} = \frac{30 \text{ ml} \times 1.5 \text{ oz}}{1 \text{ oz}}$$

$$\text{X} = 45 \text{ ml}$$

2. To convert this dosage to tablespoons, follow the same steps, using the fraction method and the conversion factor 1 Tbs = 15 ml:

- Set up a fraction with the conversion factor:

$$\frac{1 \text{ Tbs}}{15 \text{ ml}}$$

▪ Set up a fraction with the unknown household quantity:

$$\frac{X \text{ Tbs}}{45 \text{ ml}}$$

▪ Use these fractions in a proportion:

$$\frac{X \text{ Tbs}}{45 \text{ ml}} = \frac{1 \text{ Tbs}}{15 \text{ ml}}$$

▪ Solve for X by cross multiplying:

$$X \text{ Tbs} \times 15 \text{ ml} = 45 \text{ ml} \times 1 \text{ Tbs}$$

$$X = \frac{4.5 \text{ ml} \times 1 \text{ Tbs}}{15 \text{ ml}}$$

$$X = 3 \text{ Tbs}$$

Determining the number of tablets or capsules to administer

Most tablets, capsules, and similar dosage forms are available in a few strengths only. Therefore, the nurse frequently needs to administer more than 1 tablet, or ½ of a scored tablet. Breaking an unscored tablet in portions smaller than halves usually does not yield an accurate dose. Similarly, breaking a capsule in half usually results in significant loss of medication. Some oral preparations should not be opened, broken, scored, or crushed since this would change the drug's action. (See Chapter 7, Other Considerations.) If a dose smaller than ½ of a scored tablet or any portion of an unscored tablet or capsule is needed, try to substitute a commercially available solution or suspension or one that is prepared by the pharmacist.

Calculating the number of tablets or capsules to administer lends itself to the use of ratios and proportions. To do this, use the four-step process described earlier.

Patient situations

1. A drug order calls for propranolol 100 mg P.O. q.i.d., but the only available form of propranolol is 40-mg tablets. How many tablets must you administer?

▪ Set up the first ratio with the known tablet strength:

40 mg:1 tab

▪ Set up the second ratio with the desired dose and the unknown number of tablets:

100 mg:X tab

- Use these ratios in a proportion:

$$40 \text{ mg}:1 \text{ tab} :: 100 \text{ mg}:X \text{ tab}$$

- Solve for X by applying the principle that the product of the means equals the product of the extremes:

$$1 \text{ tab} \times 100 \text{ mg} = 40 \text{ mg} \times X \text{ tab}$$

$$X = \frac{1 \text{ tab} \times 100 \text{ m\cancel{g}}}{40 \text{ m\cancel{g}}}$$

$$X = 2\frac{1}{2} \text{ tab}$$

2. A patient takes half of a 0.25-mg tablet of digoxin every morning. What is the equivalent dosage in milligrams?

- Set up a fraction with the known tablet strength:

$$\frac{0.25 \text{ mg}}{1 \text{ tab}}$$

- Set up a fraction with the unknown milligram amount and the dose the patient takes:

$$\frac{X \text{ mg}}{0.5 \text{ tab}}$$

- Use these fractions in an equation, keeping similar terms in the same order on each side of the equal sign:

$$\frac{X \text{ mg}}{0.5 \text{ tab}} = \frac{0.25 \text{ mg}}{1 \text{ tab}}$$

- Solve for X by cross multiplying:

$$X \text{ mg} \times 1 \text{ tab} = 0.5 \text{ tab} \times 0.25 \text{ mg}$$

$$X = \frac{0.5 \text{ ta\cancel{b}} \times 0.25 \text{ mg}}{1 \text{ ta\cancel{b}}}$$

$$X = 0.125 \text{ mg}$$

3. Aspirin is available as 5-gr tablets. You receive an order to administer gr $\bar{x}$ q4h. How many tablets must you give?

- Set up a ratio with the known tablet strength:

$$1 \text{ tab}:5 \text{ gr}$$

- Set up a ratio with the unknown number of tablets and the desired dose:

$$X \text{ tab}:10 \text{ gr}$$

- Use the ratios in a proportion:

$$1 \text{ tab}:5 \text{ gr} :: X \text{ tabs}:10 \text{ gr}$$

■ Solve for X by applying the principle that the product of the means equals the product of the extremes:

$$5 \text{ gr} \times X \text{ tab} = 1 \text{ tab} \times 10 \text{ gr}$$

$$X = \frac{1 \text{ tab} \times 10 \text{ g\hspace{-0.5em}\diagup r}}{5 \text{ g\hspace{-0.5em}\diagup r}}$$

$$X = 2 \text{ tab}$$

Determining the amount of solution to administer

Nurses frequently need to administer medications in liquid form, either suspensions or elixirs. Calculating the amount of solution to administer can be done using either the ratio or the fraction method. To do so, use a four-step process similar to the one described for determining the number of capsules or tablets to administer:

1. Set up a ratio or fraction with the known solution strength.

2. Set up a ratio or fraction with the unknown quantity.

3. Use these ratios or fractions in a proportion.

4. Solve for X, either by applying the principle that the product of the means equals the product of the extremes (if the ratio approach is used) or by cross multiplying (if the fraction method is used).

Patient situations

1. A patient is to receive 750 mg of amoxicillin oral suspension. The label reads *AMOXICILLIN (Amoxicillin Trihydrate) 250 mg/ 5 ml. Bottle contains 100 ml.* How many milliliters of amoxicillin solution should the patient receive?

■ Set up a fraction with the known solution strength:

$$\frac{5 \text{ ml}}{250 \text{ mg}}$$

■ Set up a fraction with the unknown quantity:

$$\frac{X \text{ ml}}{750 \text{ mg}}$$

■ Set up the proportion:

$$\frac{X \text{ ml}}{750 \text{ mg}} = \frac{5 \text{ ml}}{250 \text{ mg}}$$

■ Solve for X by cross multiplying:

$$X \text{ ml} \times 250 \text{ mg} = 750 \text{ mg} \times 5 \text{ ml}$$

$$X = \frac{3,750 \text{ ml}}{250}$$

$$X = 15 \text{ ml}$$

2. Oxacillin suspension for oral administration contains 250 mg/5 ml. Based on this information from the drug label, calculate the volume needed to administer a 300-mg dose, using the ratio and proportion method:

■ Set up the ratios of the known and unknown solution strengths:

$$250 \text{ mg}:5 \text{ ml} :: 300 \text{ mg}:X \text{ ml}$$

■ Solve for X by multiplying the means and the extremes:

$$5 \text{ ml} \times 300 \text{ mg} = 250 \text{ mg} \times X \text{ ml}$$

$$X = \frac{5 \text{ ml} \times 300 \text{ m\cancel{g}}}{250 \text{ m\cancel{g}}}$$

$$X = 6 \text{ ml}$$

Determining the number of suppositories to administer

Nurses commonly administer medications in suppository form. This method is useful for patients who cannot take medications orally. You can calculate the number of suppositories to administer by using either the ratio or the fraction method already described for capsules, tablets, and solutions.

Although the physician usually orders drugs in the dosage provided by one suppository, two suppositories occasionally are needed to provide the ordered amount of medication. If you calculate that more than one is needed, you should recheck the calculations and then have another nurse perform the calculations. You should also contact the pharmacy to find out whether the medicated suppository is available in other dosages. If more than two suppositories are needed to provide one dose, contact the physician.

Teaching the patient about the purpose of the medications he is receiving is especially important when the medication is in suppository form. Many patients, for instance, presume that suppositories are given solely to promote bowel evacuation; in trying to comply with the presumed treatment, they move their bowels, thus expelling the suppository and receiving little if any medication.

Patient situations

1. The physician's order reads *Tylenol supp. gr $\bar{x}$ q4h p.r.n. temp. > 101° F.* The package label states that each suppository contains 10 grains of Tylenol. How many suppositories must you administer?

■ Set up the proportion:

$$X \text{ supp}:10 \text{ gr} :: 1 \text{ supp}:10 \text{ gr}$$

■ Solve for X:

$$X \text{ supp} \times 10 \text{ gr} = 10 \text{ gr} \times 1 \text{ supp}$$

$$X = \frac{10 \text{ gr} \times 1 \text{ supp}}{10 \text{ gr}}$$

$$X = 1 \text{ supp}$$

2. A child is to receive 60 mg of pentobarbital via suppository. The package label reads *NEMBUTAL SODIUM SUPPOSITORIES (pentobarbital sodium suppositories).* Each suppository contains 60 mg of pentobarbital sodium. How many suppositories should you administer?

■ Set up the proportion:

$$\frac{X \text{ supp}}{60 \text{ mg}} = \frac{1 \text{ supp}}{60 \text{ mg}}$$

■ Solve for X:

$$X \text{ supp} \times 60 \text{ mg} = 60 \text{ mg} \times 1 \text{ supp}$$

$$X = \frac{60 \text{ mg} \times 1 \text{ supp}}{60 \text{ mg}}$$

$$X = 1 \text{ supp}$$

Suppose that, in the above example, each suppository contains 30 mg of pentobarbital sodium. How many suppositories should you give to the patient?

■ Set up the proportion:

$$\frac{X \text{ supp}}{60 \text{ mg}} = \frac{1 \text{ supp}}{30 \text{ mg}}$$

■ Solve for X:

$$X \text{ supp} \times 30 \text{ mg} = 60 \text{ mg} \times 1 \text{ supp}$$

$$X = \frac{60 \text{ mg} \times 1 \text{ supp}}{30 \text{ mg}}$$

$$X = 2 \text{ supp}$$

Because more than one Nembutal suppository is needed, you recheck the calculations and also have another nurse perform the calculations. Next, after again determining that two suppositories should be given and noting that 60 mg is a safe dose of Nembutal for a child, you would contact the pharmacy. The pharmacist would be able to tell you that Nembutal is available in suppositories of 30, 60, 120, and 200 mg. By using a 60-mg suppository, you would be able to give the child one rather than two.

If, in the same example, the patient was to receive 30 mg of pentobarbital and each suppository contained 60 mg, how many suppositories would you give to the patient?

- Set up the proportion:

$$\frac{\text{X supp}}{30 \text{ mg}} = \frac{1 \text{ supp}}{60 \text{ mg}}$$

- Solve for X:

$$\text{X supp} \times 60 \text{ mg} = 30 \text{ mg} \times 1 \text{ supp}$$

$$\text{X} = \frac{30 \text{ mg} \times 1 \text{ supp}}{60 \text{ mg}}$$

$$\text{X} = 0.5 \text{ supp}$$

Because less than one Nembutal suppository is needed, you recheck the calculations and also have another nurse perform the calculations. Rather than give half of the available 60-mg suppository, you contact the pharmacy to order Nembutal in a 30-mg suppository, if available.

COMPUTATION OF DOSAGES REQUIRING TWO STEPS

Most dosage calculations require more than one simple equation. Medications may be ordered in one system of measurement but may be available in tablet, capsule, or liquid form in another system of measurement. When these situations occur, you must convert from one system to another (see "Converting Between Measurement Systems," page 78, for a review) and then determine the number of capsules or tablets or the amount of solution to administer (see "Determining the Number of Tablets or Capsules to Administer," page 83, and "Determining the Amount of Solution to Administer," page 85, for a review). This section describes how to perform complete dosage calculations based on drug order and drug label information, using the ratio or fraction method.

Basic guidelines

Use the following guidelines to determine the number of capsules or tablets or the amount of solution to be given to the patient (either the ratio or fraction method for dosage calculations may be used for these calculations):

1. Read the drug order thoroughly, paying close attention to decimal places and zeros.
2. Convert the dose from the system in which it is ordered to the system in which it is available.
3. Calculate the number of capsules or tablets or the amount of solution needed to obtain the desired dose.
The following patient situations illustrate various dosage calculations from start to finish.

Patient situations

1. The physician's order states *Lithium carbonate gr $\bar{x}$ p.o. t.i.d.* The drug label states *Lithium Carbonate USP 300 milligrams/ capsule.* How many capsules should you give to the patient for one dose?

■ Knowing that gr $\bar{x}$ = 10 grains, you first convert the dose from the system in which it is ordered to the system in which it is available, using the following proportion:

$$\frac{X \text{ mg}}{10 \text{ gr}} = \frac{60 \text{ mg}}{1 \text{ gr}}$$

■ Solve for X:

$$X \text{ mg} \times 1 \text{ gr} = 10 \text{ gr} \times 60 \text{ mg}$$

$$X = \frac{10 \text{ gr} \times 60 \text{ mg}}{1 \text{ gr}}$$

$$X = 600 \text{ mg}$$

■ In the second portion of the calculations, you determine the number of capsules to administer, as follows:

$$\frac{X \text{ cap}}{600 \text{ mg}} = \frac{1 \text{ cap}}{300 \text{ mg}}$$

■ Solve for X:

$$X \text{ cap} \times 300 \text{ mg} = 600 \text{ mg} \times 1 \text{ cap}$$

$$X = \frac{600 \text{ mg} \times 1 \text{ cap}}{300 \text{ mg}}$$

$$X = 2 \text{ cap}$$

2. A drug order calls for digoxin pediatric elixir 0.125 mg P.O. once daily. To determine how much elixir to administer, read the label on the bottle, which contains 50 mcg/ml, and begin the calculation with a conversion so that both terms will be expressed in the same units of measure.

▪ Convert milligrams to micrograms, using the conversion factor of 1 mg = 1,000 mcg:

$$1 \text{ mg}:1,000 \text{ mcg} :: 0.125 \text{ mg}:X \text{ mcg}$$

$$1,000 \text{ mcg} \times 0.125 \text{ mg} = 1 \text{ mg} \times X \text{ mcg}$$

$$X = \frac{1,000 \text{ mcg} \times 0.125 \text{ m\!\!\!/g}}{1 \text{ m\!\!\!/g}}$$

$$X = 125 \text{ mcg}$$

▪ Once both terms appear in the same unit of measure, you can calculate the volume of elixir to administer:

$$50 \text{ mcg}:1 \text{ ml} :: 125 \text{ mcg}:X \text{ ml}$$

$$1 \text{ ml} \times 125 \text{ mcg} = 50 \text{ mcg} \times X \text{ ml}$$

$$X = \frac{1 \text{ ml} \times 125 \text{ m\!c\!g}}{50 \text{ m\!c\!g}}$$

$$X = 2.5 \text{ ml}$$

This drug comes with a special dropper calibrated in mcg and ml. Read the calibration marks carefully when administering this drug because it has a narrow therapeutic margin.

3. A patient is to receive 450 mg of aminophylline. The label states *Aminophylline Suppositories USP*. Each suppository contains 7½ grains. How many suppositories should the patient receive?

▪ First, convert the dose from the system in which it is ordered to the system in which it is available, using the following proportion:

$$\frac{X \text{ gr}}{450 \text{ mg}} = \frac{1 \text{ gr}}{60 \text{ mg}}$$

▪ Solve for X:

$$X \text{ gr} \times 60 \text{ mg} = 450 \text{ mg} \times 1 \text{ gr}$$

$$X = \frac{450 \text{ m\!\!\!/g} \times 1 \text{ gr}}{60 \text{ m\!\!\!/g}}$$

$$X = 7.5 \text{ gr}$$

▪ In the second portion of the calculations, determine the number of suppositories to administer, as follows:

$$\frac{X \text{ supp}}{7.5 \text{ gr}} = \frac{1 \text{ supp}}{7.5 \text{ gr}}$$

▪ Solve for X:

$$X \text{ supp} \times 7.5 \text{ gr} = 7.5 \text{ gr} \times 1 \text{ supp}$$

$$X = \frac{7.5 \text{ gr} \times 1 \text{ supp}}{7.5 \text{ gr}}$$

$$X = 1 \text{ supp}$$

"Desired-over-have" and "ordered-available" approaches

Some individuals prefer to think of drug calculations in terms of what is desired or ordered for the patient and what one has available. The desired-over-have and ordered-available approaches use essentially the same proportions for converting between measurement systems as those already described, except that the ordered-available approach incorporates two steps into one equation.

The desired-over-have approach

The desired-over-have approach uses a fraction to express known and unknown quantities:

$$\frac{\text{Desired units}}{\text{Have units (X)}} = \text{Equivalent} \left(\frac{\text{Same units as Desired}}{\text{Same units as Have}} \right)$$

Patient situation

Ten grains of aspirin are ordered (desired), and 300-mg tablets are available (what you have). How many tablets must you administer?

▪ First, convert between systems from what is desired (grains) to what you have on hand (milligrams):

$$\frac{10 \text{ gr}}{X \text{ mg}} = \frac{1 \text{ gr}}{60 \text{ mg}}$$

▪ Solve for X:

$$X \text{ mg} \times 1 \text{ gr} = 10 \text{ gr} \times 60 \text{ mg}$$

$$X = \frac{10 \text{ gr} \times 60 \text{ mg}}{1 \text{ gr}}$$

$$X = 600 \text{ mg}$$

■ Next, calculate the number of tablets to administer to provide one 600-mg dose, using the proportion:

$$\frac{X \text{ tab desired}}{1 \text{ tab have}} = \frac{600 \text{ mg desired}}{300 \text{ mg have}}$$

■ Solve for X:

$$X \text{ tab} \times 300 \text{ mg} = 1 \text{ tab} \times 600 \text{ mg}$$

$$X = \frac{1 \text{ tab} \times 600 \text{ mg}}{300 \text{ mg}}$$

$$X = 2 \text{ tab}$$

The ordered-available approach

Unlike the desired-over-have-approach, the ordered-available approach uses only one equation to convert between systems of measurement and to calculate the amount of medication to administer. However, if you misplace any part of the equation (such as placing a quantity in the numerator that should be in the denominator), the error may not be immediately apparent, leading to significant errors in calculation. Although the two-step desired-over-have approach may take slightly more time, the ratios or fractions used in each step can be quickly checked to ensure correct placement of the units of measure, which helps prevent errors.

The ordered-available approach is presented here for those who wish to learn it:

$$X \text{ tab} = \text{ordered dose} \times \text{conversion factor} \times \frac{\text{available amount of dosage form}}{\text{quantity of drug per dosage form}}$$

Patient situation

The physician orders 5 grains of ferrous sulfate, and 300-mg tablets are available. How many tablets should you administer?

■ Using the ordered-available approach:

$$X \text{ tab} = 5 \text{ gr} \times \frac{60 \text{ mg}}{1 \text{ gr}} \times \frac{1 \text{ tab}}{300 \text{ mg}}$$

■ Solve for X:

$$X \text{ tab} = \frac{5 \text{ gr} \times 60 \text{ mg} \times 1 \text{ tab}}{1 \text{ gr} \times 300 \text{ mg}}$$

$$X = \frac{300 \text{ tab}}{300}$$

$$X = 1 \text{ tab}$$

PRACTICE PROBLEMS

Tablets

The answers to these problems follow on page 101.

1. The physician orders Hexadrol 8 mg p.o. The label on the bottle is:

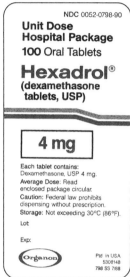

NDC 0052-0798-90

**Unit Dose
Hospital Package**
100 Oral Tablets

Hexadrol®
**(dexamethasone
tablets, USP)**

4 mg

Each tablet contains:
Dexamethasone, USP 4 mg.
Average Dose: Read
enclosed package circular.
Caution: Federal law prohibits
dispensing without prescription.
Storage: Not exceeding 30°C (86°F).

Lot:

Exp:

Organon

Ptd in USA
5308148
798 SS 7/88

You would administer _____ tablets.

2. The physician orders Cardizem 90 mg p.o. The label on the bottle is:

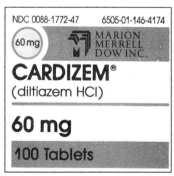

NDC 0088-1772-47   6505-01-146-4174

60 mg

MARION
MERRELL
DOW INC.

CARDIZEM®
(diltiazem HCl)

60 mg

100 Tablets

You would administer _____ tablets.

3. The physician orders Coumadin 7.5 mg p.o. The label on the bottle is:

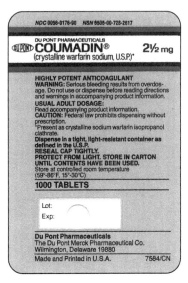

You would administer _____ tablets.

4. The physician orders Norpramin 50 mg p.o. The label on the bottle is:

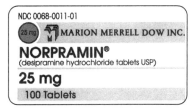

You would administer _____ tablets.

5. If a drug order calls for 30 mg of propanolol, but the only available form is 20-mg tablets, you would administer

_____ .

6. If hydroxyzine hydrochloride is available in 10-mg tablets but the drug order calls for a 20-mg dose, you would administer _____ .

7. If chlorothiazide is available in 500-mg tablets but the drug order calls for a 750-mg dose, you would administer

_____.

8. If Hexadrol is available in 1.5-mg tablets but the drug order calls for a 6-mg dose, you would administer

_____.

9. If Cylert is available in 37.5-mg tablets but the drug order calls for a 56.25-mg dose, you would administer

_____.

10. If Synthroid is available in 100-mcg tablets but the drug order calls for a 250-mcg dose, you would administer

_____.

11. If Cardizem is available in 30-mg tablets but the drug order calls for a 60-mg dose, you would administer

_____.

12. If Zyloprim is available in 100-mg tablets but the drug order calls for a 300-mg dose, you would administer

_____.

13. If Tenormin is available in 50-mg tablets but the drug order calls for a 100-mg dose, you would administer

_____ .

14. If spironolactone is available in 25-mg tablets but the drug order calls for a 150-mg dose, you would administer

_____ .

15. If Coumadin is available in 2.5-mg tablets but the drug order calls for a 5-mg dose, you would administer

_____ .

16. If desipramine hydrochloride is available in 25-mg tablets but the drug order calls for a 100-mg dose, you would administer

_____ .

17. If propranolol hydrochloride is available in 60-mg tablets but the drug order calls for a 90-mg dose, you would administer

_____ .

18. If bisacodyl is available in 5-mg tablets but the drug order calls for a 20-mg dose, you would administer

_____ .

19. If verapamil hydrochloride is available in 80-mg tablets but the drug order calls for a 120-mg dose, you would administer

_____ .

20. If digoxin is available in 0.25-mg tablets but the drug order calls for an initial 0.375-mg dose, you would administer

_____ .

Enteral liquids
The answers to these problems follow on page 102.

1. The physician orders Keflex 250 mg p.o. The label on the bottle is:

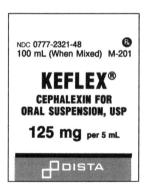

You would administer _____ ml.

2. The physician orders Nystatin 200,000 U p.o. The label on the bottle is:

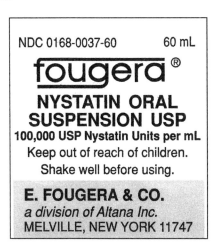

NDC 0168-0037-60   60 mL

fougera®

NYSTATIN ORAL SUSPENSION USP

100,000 USP Nystatin Units per mL

Keep out of reach of children.
Shake well before using.

E. FOUGERA & CO.

a division of Altana Inc.
MELVILLE, NEW YORK 11747

You would administer _____ ml.

3. The physician orders Ceclor 125 mg p.o. for a child. The label on the bottle is:

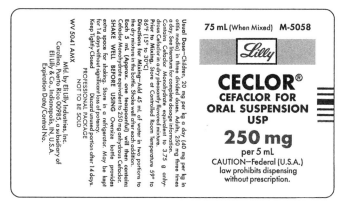

75 mL (When Mixed)   M-5058

Lilly

CECLOR®
CEFACLOR FOR
ORAL SUSPENSION
USP

250 mg
per 5 mL
CAUTION—Federal (U.S.A.)
law prohibits dispensing
without prescription.

Usual Dose—Children, 20 mg per kg a day (40 mg per kg in otitis media) in three divided doses. Adults, 250 mg three times a day. See literature for complete dosage information. Contains Cefaclor Monohydrate equivalent to 3.75 g anhydrous Cefaclor in a dry pleasantly flavored mixture.

Prior to Mixing, Store at Controlled Room temperature 59° to 86°F (15° to 30°C)

Directions for Mixing—Add 45 mL of water in two portions to the dry mixture in the bottle. Shake well after each addition. Each 5 mL (Approx. one teaspoonful) will then contain Cefaclor Monohydrate equivalent to 250 mg anhydrous Cefaclor.

SHAKE WELL BEFORE USING. Oversize bottle provides extra space for shaking. Store in a refrigerator. May be kept for 14 days without significant loss of potency. Discard unused portion after 14 days.

Keep Tightly Closed

PROFESSIONAL PACKAGE
NOT TO BE SOLD

Mfd. by Eli Lilly Industries, Inc.
Carolina, Puerto Rico 00985, a subsidiary of
Eli Lilly & Co., Indianapolis, IN, U.S.A.
Expiration Date/Control No.

WV 5041 AMX

You would administer _____ ml.

4. If ampicillin is available as an oral suspension with 125 mg in every 5 ml but the drug order calls for 250 mg, you would administer _____ .

5. If Kay Ciel is available for oral replacement as 20 mEq/15 ml but the drug order calls for 10 mEq, you would administer

_____ .

6. To administer a 200-mg dose of amoxicillin, you would have to give _____ ml of a 250 mg/5ml amoxicillin suspension.

7. Docusate comes in 250-mg capsules and in a 150 mg/15 ml liquid. You would have to give _____ ml of docusate liquid to give the same dose as in 1 capsule.

8. For an elderly patient who cannot swallow a 160-mg furosemide tablet, you could administer _____ ml of furosemide in a 10 mg/ml liquid form.

9. A patient is to receive Elixophyllin 200 mg p.o. The label on the bottle indicates a concentration of 100 mg/5ml. You would administer _____ ml.

10. A patient is to receive Amoxil 250 mg p.o. q8h. Amoxil is available in a 150-ml bottle, with a concentration of 250 mg/5 ml. This bottle will provide _____ doses and will last _____ days.

Converting between systems: Weight
The answers to these problems follow on page 102.

1. If an infant weighs 3,409 g at birth, you would tell the mother that her baby weighs _____ lb,

_____ oz.

2. If a patient weighs 250 lbs, his weight in kg is

_____ .

3. If a patient weighs 60 kg on admission and his wife says he normally weighs 165 lb, he has lost _____ lb.

4. If a baby doubles her 3,000-g birth weight by age 5 months, she will weigh _____ lb at that time.

5. If a child weighs 20 kg, her weight in pounds is

_____.

Converting between systems: Tablets and capsules
The answers to these problems follow on page 102.

1. If a drug order calls for gr ½ of phenobarbital and your supply is in 32-mg tablets, you would administer

_____.

2. If a drug order calls for 600 mg of acetaminophen and you have gr v̄/tablet, you would administer _____.

3. If a drug order calls for quinidine sulfate gr v̄ and the tablets are identified as 325 mg per tablet, you would administer _____.

4. If a drug order calls for Gantrisin gr XV and the tablets are identified as 500 mg per tablet, you would administer

_____.

5. A patient is to receive Quinaglute Dura-Tabs gr v̄ g12h. You have on hand tablets marked 324 mg. You will administer _____ tablets.

6. The physician prescribes chloral hydrate gr XV h.s. You have on hand 500-mg capsules. You will administer _____ capsules.

7. A patient is to receive Nembutal gr īss h.s. You have on hand 50-mg capsules. You will administer _____ capsules.

8. The physician prescribes Synthroid 150 mcg as a daily replacement dose. The pharmacy sends you 0.3-mg tablets. You will administer _____ tablets.

9. An adult patient with myxedema is to receive 2 months of therapy with dessicated thyroid at a daily dosage of gr $\overline{\text{ii}}$. The tablets supplied are labeled 32 mg. You will administer _____ tablets per day.

10. You must give _____ 250-mg procainamide capsules to administer a 750-mg dose.

Converting between systems: Enteral liquids

The answers to these problems follow on page 103.

1. If a drug order calls for atropine sulfate 0.4 mg and you have gr$^1/_{150}$/ml, you would administer _____.

2. If a patient has been receiving 10 ml of Maalox in the hospital and is to continue on the same dosage at home, you would tell him to take _____ tsp.

3. If a drug order calls for Kaon Elixir 20 mEq and the preparation contains 20 mEq/15 ml, you would tell the patient to take _____ Tbs at home.

4. If a patient has been taking 2 Tbs of milk of magnesia at home to prevent constipation, you would request an order for _____ ml to continue the same dosage.

5. If a patient tells you he has been taking 2 tsp of Tagamet with each meal and the drug contains 300 mg/5 ml, he has been receiving _____ mg each dose.

6. A child, age 7, is to receive Mandelamine gr $\overline{\text{viiss}}$ q.i.d. The oral suspension supplied contains 0.25 G/5 ml. You will administer _____ ml per dose.

7. A 170-lb male patient is to receive ethambutol hydrochloride 15 mg/kg daily to treat tuberculosis. The drug is available in 100 and 400-mg tablets. You will administer _____ .

8. A 33-lb child is to receive Coly-Mycin S 15 mg/kg/day in three divided doses. The oral suspension on hand contains 25 mg/5 ml. You will administer _____ ml per dose.

9. To administer a 200-mg dose of amoxicillin, you would have to give _____ ml of a 250 mg/5ml amoxicillin suspension.

10. A teaspoon of a solution labeled potassium 20 m/Eq/15 ml contains _____ mEq of potassium.

ANSWERS TO PRACTICE PROBLEMS

Tablets

1. 2 tablets
2. 1.5 tablets
3. 3 tablets
4. 2 tablets
5. 1.5 tablets
6. 2 tablets
7. 1.5 tablets
8. 4 tablets
9. 1.5 tablets
10. 2.5 tablets
11. 2 tablets
12. 3 tablets
13. 2 tablets
14. 6 tablets
15. 2 tablets
16. 4 tablets
17. 1.5 tablets
18. 4 tablets
19. 1.5 tablets
20. 1.5 tablets

Enteral liquids

1. 10 ml
2. 2 ml
3. 2.5 ml
4. 10 ml
5. 7.5 ml
6. 4 ml
7. 25 ml
8. 16 ml
9. 10 ml
10. 30 doses, 10 days

Converting between systems: Weight

1. 7 lb, 8 oz
2. 113.6 kg
3. 33 lb
4. 13.2 lb
5. 44 lb

Converting between systems: Tablets and capusles

1. 1 tablet
2. 2 tablets
3. 1 tablet
4. 2 tablets
5. 1 tablet
6. 2 capsules
7. 2 capsules
8. ½ tablet
9. 4 tablets
10. 3 capsules

Converting between systems: Enteral liquids

1. 1 ml
2. 2 tsp
3. 1 Tbs

4. 30 ml

5. 600 mg

6. 10 ml

7. three 400-mg tablets (1,200 mg)

8. 15 ml

9. 4 ml

10. 6.67 mEq

CALCULATING PARENTERAL DRUG DOSAGES

P arenteral medications are drugs that are introduced into the body by a route other than the gastrointestinal tract. Commonly thought of as injectables, parenteral drugs may be administered via the intravenous (I.V.), intramuscular (I.M.), subcutaneous (S.C.), or intrathecal routes.

When performing dosage calculations for parenteral drug administration, you'll need to be aware of special considerations. For example, you may need to determine a solution's strength and flow rate based on information given in the physician's order. This chapter reviews calculations relating to parenteral solution preparation, insulin administration, administration of I.V. fluid and other parenteral products, infusion pumps, and patient-controlled analgesia.

ADMINISTRATION OF PREPARED LIQUIDS

The methods for computing drug dosages for prepared liquids (see Chapter 4, Calculating Enteral Drug Dosages) can be used for oral or parenteral routes. The label on a prepared liquid indicates the drug's concentration, usually expressed as milligrams per milliliter or units per milliliter.

Parenteral liquids may be administered through syringes (see *Syringes and needles*). In some cases, the syringes are prefilled, which reduces medication preparation time, decreases medication errors, and simplifies recording the amount of drug used. Narcotics commonly are supplied in this form.

The following patient situation shows how to determine the dosage of a liquid medication to be administered parenterally.

SYRINGES AND NEEDLES

SYRINGES

Standard syringes, available in 3-, 5-, 10-, 25-, 30-, 35-, and 50-ml sizes, are used to administer various medications in numerous settings. Each syringe consists of a plunger, barrel, hub, needle, and dead space. The dead space holds the fluid remaining in the syringe and needle when the plunger is completely depressed. Some syringes, such as insulin syringes, do not have dead space areas.

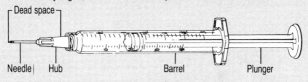

Dead space · Needle | Hub · Barrel · Plunger

The **insulin syringe** has an attached 25-gauge (25G) needle and no dead space. The syringe is divided into units rather than milliliters for measurement. This syringe should be used only for insulin administration.

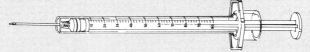

The **tuberculin syringe** holds up to 1 ml of medication. Used most frequently for intradermal injections, it is also used to administer small volumes of medication, such as might be required in pediatric and intensive care units.

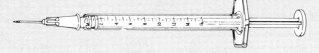

A **prefilled syringe** reduces medication preparation time and decreases the likelihood of medication errors.

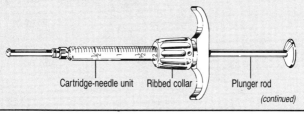

Cartridge-needle unit · Ribbed collar · Plunger rod

(continued)

SYRINGES AND NEEDLES *(continued)*

NEEDLES

When choosing a needle, consider its gauge (inside diameter), bevel (angle at which the needle tip opens), and length (from tip to hub). Remember: The smaller the gauge, the larger the diameter.

Needleless needles are 18G-, 1-in (2.5 cm-) needles used for administration into I.V. lines or heparin flush caps. They reduce the risk of needle sticks and their sequelae.

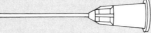

Intradermal needles are ⅜ in to ⅝ in (1 to 1.5 cm) long, usually have short bevels, and are 25G in diameter.

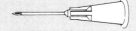

Subcutaneous needles are ½ in to ⅞ in (1.3 to 2 cm) long, have medium bevels, and are 25G to 23G in diameter.

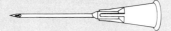

Intramuscular needles are 1 in to 3 in (2.5 to 7.5 cm) long, have medium bevels, and are 23G to 18G in diameter.

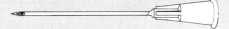

Intravenous needles are 1 in to 3 in long, have long bevels, and are 25G to 14G in diameter.

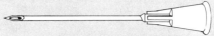

Filter needles, which should not be used for injection, are 1½ in (4 cm) long, have medium bevels, and are 20G in diameter. Microscopic pieces of rubber or glass may enter the solution when the nurse punctures the diaphragm of a vial with a needle or snaps open an ampule. The nurse can use a filter needle with a screening device contained within the hub to remove minute particles of foreign material from a solution.

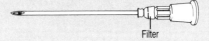

Filter

SYRINGES AND NEEDLES *(continued)*

NEEDLES *(continued)*

A **closed system device** comes with the needle in place. These devices have either a plunger attached (prefilled syringe) or a cartridge to be inserted into a barrel with a plunger attached (cartridge-needle unit, as shown below). Emergency drugs, such as atropine and lidocaine, are available in prefilled syringes. Narcotic analgesics, heparin, and injectable vitamins are available in cartridge-needle units.

To prepare the prefilled syringe, hold the medication chamber in one hand and the syringe and needle in the other. Flip the protective caps off both ends. Insert the medication chamber into the syringe section. Remove the needle cap and expel any air in the system.

To prepare the cartridge-needle for use, insert a cartridge into the syringe. Twist the barrel until it is engaged. Then, insert the plunger and twist until the barrel rotates in the syringe. Remove the needle cap and purge the device of air and any extra medication.

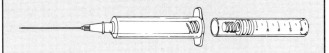

Patient situation

The physician orders 75 mg of Demerol. The available solution contains 100 mg/ml. You need to calculate the number of milliliters of Demerol solution to administer.

■ Using the fraction method, set up the proportion:

$$\frac{75 \text{ mg}}{\text{X ml}} = \frac{100 \text{ mg}}{1 \text{ ml}}$$

■ Solve for X:

$$\text{X ml} \times 100 \text{ mg} = 75 \text{ mg} \times 1 \text{ ml}$$

$$\text{X} = \frac{75 \text{ ml}}{100}$$

$$\text{X} = 0.75 \text{ ml}$$

You should give 0.75 or ¾ ml of the solution.

■ Should you need to know the number of minims that would deliver the same dose, you can use the ratio method and set up the following proportion:

$$\text{X M}_x\text{:}0.75 \text{ ml} :: 15 \text{ M}_x\text{:}1 \text{ ml}$$

■ Solve for X:

$$X \, M_x \times 1 \text{ ml} = 0.75 \text{ ml} \times 15 \, M_x$$
$$X = 12 \, M_x$$

Twelve minims, or 0.75 ml, would contain the 75 mg of Demerol ordered.

ADMINISTRATION OF INSULIN

To handle the special needs of diabetic patients, you need to know about the different types of insulin and insulin orders, the different types of insulin syringes and their proper use, and the procedures for safely handling and drawing up various types of insulin.

Insulin therapy

Insulin, a potent hormone produced by the pancreas, regulates carbohydrate metabolism, which is reflected in blood glucose levels. An absolute or relative lack of insulin results in diabetes.

Two major types of diabetes exist: insulin-dependent diabetes mellitus (type I), which usually is diagnosed before age 20 and requires long-term insulin therapy; and noninsulin-dependent diabetes mellitus (type II), which usually is diagnosed after age 40 and controlled by diet therapy and oral hypoglycemic agents, although exogenous insulin may be used to stabilize blood glucose levels. For either type of diabetes, physicians can prescribe insulin that is commercially available from several sources.

Some insulins are identical to human insulin and are produced by enzymatic conversion of pork insulin or by recombinant DNA techniques. Others are derived from bovine (beef) or porcine (pork) pancreas and differ from human insulin by only two amino acids. (However, manufacturers have removed many purified beef insulins and insulin zinc suspensions from the market because of their limited use among diabetic patients.) Regardless of product type, insulin dosages must be calculated and administered carefully. They must be administered parenterally: intravenously when immediate onset of action is desired and subcutaneously when a slower onset and more sustained duration of action are desired. When regular insulin is added to a large-volume I.V.

INSULIN LABELING

The many types of insulin are not all interchangeable, and you must read the labels carefully. The patient's response is related to both insulin type (regular, NPH) and derivation (pork, human). *Thus, changing a patient's insulin may cause widely fluctuating variations in blood glucose levels.* Insulin labels tell you what you need to know to administer the correct type and concentration.

- Lente human insulin zinc suspension (semisynthetic)
- Lente purified pork insulin zinc suspension USP
- NPH human insulin isophane suspension (semi-synthetic)
- NPH purified pork isophane insulin suspension USP
- 70% NPH, human insulin isophane suspension and 30% regular, human insulin injection (semisynthetic)
- Regular human insulin injection USP (semisynthetic)
- Regular insulin, insulin injection USP (pork)
- Regular purified pork insulin injection USP

infusion, some of it binds to the tubing and container. In some situations, albumin may be added to the infusion; albumin binds with the insulin and prevents it from binding elsewhere.

Several kinds of insulin are available. (For examples of the types of insulin and labeling information on insulin vials, see *Insulin labeling.*) The various insulin preparations have been modified by combination with larger insoluble protein molecules to slow absorption and prolong activity. Thus, they differ in onset, peak, and duration of action. Because of these differences, insulins are classified as rapid-acting, intermediate-acting, and long-acting.

Insulin doges, expressed in units (U) based on bioassay of activity, are available in several concentrations. U-100 (100 units of insulin per milliliter) is the most commonly used, "universal" concentration. U-40 (40 units of insulin per milliliter), a weaker solution, may still be used by a few older individuals. Another concentration, U-500 (500 units of insulin per milliliter), is available for the rare instances in which a patient needs an exceptionally large dose of insulin.

The insulin syringe you use must be compatible with the strength of the insulin you are administering. Thus, if 20 units of U-100 regular insulin were ordered, you would use a U-100 syringe and draw up the insulin to the 20 unit mark. (See *Insulin syringes,* page 110, for examples of the most common types.)

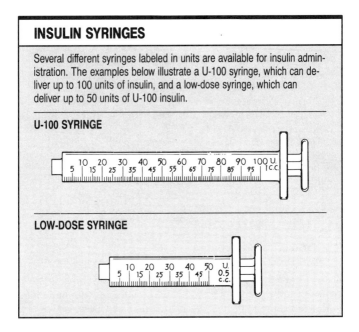

INSULIN SYRINGES

Several different syringes labeled in units are available for insulin administration. The examples below illustrate a U-100 syringe, which can deliver up to 100 units of insulin, and a low-dose syringe, which can deliver up to 50 units of U-100 insulin.

U-100 SYRINGE

LOW-DOSE SYRINGE

Reading insulin orders

When diabetes is diagnosed, the physician orders blood and urine glucose determinations, usually in a hospital where the patient's diet is controlled and around-the-clock values can be measured and blood and urine glucose baselines can be established. Based on these determinations, the physician may order small doses of rapid-acting insulin at set times, such as every 4 hours or before meals and at bedtime, for several days. After a stable 24-hour dosage has been determined, the physician may order dosage adjustments, such as one or two daily doses of intermediate-acting insulin, possibly accompanied by small doses of rapid-acting insulin.

For a newly diagnosed, ill, or unstable diabetic patient, the physician may write an order on a sliding scale, which individualizes the insulin quantities and administration times according to the patient's age, exercise and work habits, desired degree of blood glucose level control, and response to insulin preparations, as shown in this example:

Blood glucose values	Insulin dose
< 180 mg/dl	No insulin
180 to 240 mg/dl	10 units of regular insulin S.C.
241 to 400 mg/dl	20 units of regular insulin S.C.
> 400 mg/dl	Call physician for orders

Some patients may receive insulin doses based on home monitoring of blood glucose values with glucometers. In the past, patients also had their insulin doses adjusted on a sliding scale based on urine glucose values, as shown in this example:

Urine glucose values	Insulin dose
0 to 1/4%	No insulin
1/2%	10 units of regular insulin
1%	15 units of regular insulin
2%	20 units of regular insulin

Such a patient might receive additional insulin if ketones appear in the urine.

When reading insulin orders, be alert to the placement of decimal points. Some patients are extremely sensitive to insulin, requiring a dose of less than 10 units. To clarify this, a physician may write the dose with a decimal point, which may be overlooked on a line of writing and mistakenly dropped during transcription. For example, a physician may want to order 3 units of insulin and may write 3.0 units of insulin for clarity. If the decimal point is lost in transcription, the patient could receive 30 units of insulin, a tenfold dosage error. Always check doses that seem unusually large or small.

Processing insulin orders

Once insulin has been ordered, you need to draw it up and administer it. To ensure that the correct dose of the proper insulin is administered, follow this procedure:

1. Read the vial label carefully, noting the type, concentration, source, and expiration date of the insulin. Most patients receive U-100 insulin, which contains 100 units of insulin per milliliter of solution or suspension. Others may receive U-40 insulin, which is used for patients accustomed to using this concentration or those who need small doses, or U-500 insulin, which is used for patients with insulin resistance who require high doses. Patients may receive a combination of NPH and regular insulin (see *Combining NPH and regular insulin,* page 112).

COMBINING NPH AND REGULAR INSULIN

NPH and regular insulin in combination are commonly administered simultaneously. When you receive an order for this combination of drugs, draw them up into the same syringe following this procedure:

■ Read the insulin order carefully.

■ Read the vial labels carefully, noting the type, concentration, source, and expiration date of the drugs.

■ Roll the NPH vial between the palms of your hands to mix it properly.

■ Choose the appropriate syringe.

■ Clean the tops of both vials with alcohol sponges.

■ Inject air into the NPH vial equal to the amount of insulin you need to administer. Withdraw the needle and syringe, but do not withdraw any NPH insulin.

■ Now inject into the regular insulin vial an amount of air equal to the dose of regular insulin. Then invert or tilt the vial and withdraw the ordered amount of regular insulin into the syringe. (Regular insulin is drawn up first to avoid contamination by the addition of longer-acting insulin.)

■ Clean the top of the NPH vial again. Then insert into this vial the needle of the syringe containing the regular insulin and withdraw the ordered amount of the NPH insulin.

■ Mix the insulins in the syringe by pulling back slightly on the plunger and tilting the syringe back and forth.

■ Recheck the drug orders and administer and chart the medications immediately.

2. Choose the appropriate syringe. Insulin syringes are designed to measure insulin accurately. When administering U-100 insulin, use a U-100 syringe. This type of syringe is calibrated to measure up to 1 ml (100 units) of insulin in 1- or 2-unit increments. When drawing up doses of less than 50 units, use a low-dose syringe, which is calibrated in 1-unit increments. This type of syringe is particularly useful for drawing up doses of less than 20 units.

3. Withdraw the ordered amount of insulin into the syringe, using appropriate aseptic technique.

4. Recheck the insulin order and administer and chart the medication.

Patient situation

The physician's order states *20 U NPH Human Insulin s.c. q.d. (7 a.m.).* The order also calls for a blood glucose measurement daily at 3 p.m., with coverage as follows:

Blood glucose values	Insulin dose
200 mg/dl	0 units
200 to 250 mg/dl	5 units
251 to 300 mg/dl	10 units
301 to 350 mg/dl	15 units
> 350 mg/dl	Call physician for orders

If the patient's glucose level is 260 mg/dl at 3 p.m., how many units of regular human insulin would you administer?

■ Locate the patient's blood glucose level (260 mg/dl) under "Blood glucose values" in the physician's order.

■ Find the corresponding dose under "Insulin dose."
You would administer 10 units of regular human insulin S.C.

RECONSTITUTION OF A POWDER

Although the pharmacist may reconstitute powders for parenteral use, you may have to perform this task. If so, keep the following points in mind.

When reconstituting powders for injection, consult the drug label. It will give the total quantity of drug in the vial or ampule, the amount and type of diluent to add to the powder, and the strength and shelf life (expiration date) of the resulting solution. When diluent is added to a powder, the powder increases the fluid volume. For this reason, the label calls for less diluent than the total volume of the prepared solution. For example, you may have to add 1.7 ml of diluent to a vial of powdered drug to obtain a 2-ml total volume of prepared solution. Follow the directions on the drug label.

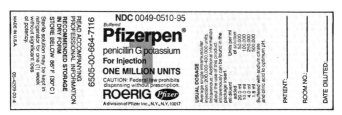

■ To determine how much solution to administer, use the manufacturer's information about the concentration of the solution. For example, if you want to administer 500 mg of a drug and the concentration of the prepared solution is 1 G (1,000 mg) per 10 ml, you can set up a fraction proportion as follows:

$$\frac{X \text{ ml}}{500 \text{ mg}} = \frac{10 \text{ ml}}{1,000 \text{ mg}}$$

■ Solve for X:

$$X \text{ ml} \times 1,000 \text{ mg} = 500 \text{ mg} \times 10 \text{ ml}$$

$$X = \frac{5,000 \text{ ml}}{1,000}$$

$$X = 5 \text{ ml}$$

■ If you prefer the ratio approach, set up the proportion as follows:

$$X \text{ ml}:500 \text{ mg} :: 10 \text{ ml}:1,000 \text{ mg}$$

■ Solve for X:

$$X \text{ ml} \times 1,000 \text{ mg} = 500 \text{ mg} \times 10 \text{ ml}$$

$$X = \frac{5,000 \text{ ml}}{1,000}$$

$$X = 5 \text{ ml}$$

By using either approach (fraction or ratio), you would calculate that 5 ml of solution must be given so the patient receives 500 mg of the drug.

Patient situation

The physician orders 500 mg of ampicillin for a patient. A 1-G vial of powdered ampicillin is available. The label states *Add 4.5 ml sterile water to yield 1 G/5 ml.* How many milliliters of reconstituted ampicillin should you give the patient?

■ First, dilute the powder according to the instructions on the label. The concentration listed on the label provides the first portion of the proportion:

$$\frac{1 \text{ G}}{5 \text{ ml}}$$

■ Next, make sure the same units of measure appear in both denominators of the proportion. In this case, the units must both be grams or milligrams. If you use milligrams and the fraction method, the proportion would be:

$$\frac{X \text{ ml}}{500 \text{ mg}} = \frac{5 \text{ ml}}{1,000 \text{ mg}}$$

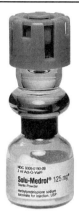

Two-chambered vial with rubber stopper

▪ Solve for X:

$$X \text{ ml} \times 1{,}000 \text{ mg} = 500 \text{ mg} \times 5 \text{ ml}$$

$$X = \frac{2{,}500 \text{ ml}}{1{,}000}$$

$$X = 2.5 \text{ ml}$$

Give 2.5 ml of the solution, which will deliver 500 mg of ampicillin.

Some medications that require reconstitution are packaged in vials that have two chambers separated by a rubber stopper (see illustration above). The upper chamber contains the diluent and the lower chamber contains the powdered drug. When you depress the top of the vial, the rubber stopper between the two chambers dislodges, allowing the diluent to flow into the lower chamber, where it can mix with the powdered drug. Then you can remove the correct amount of solution with a syringe.

ADMINISTRATION OF INTRAVENOUS FLUID

Calculations for I.V. administration typically involve determining the drip rate (the number of drops of solution that will infuse per minute) and the flow rate (the number of milliliters of solution that will infuse over a given time).

Calculating I.V. drip rates

To determine the I.V. drip rate, first set up a fraction showing the volume of infusion over the number of minutes in which that volume is to be infused. For example, if a patient is to receive 100 ml of solution within 1 hour, the fraction would be written as:

$$\frac{100 \text{ ml}}{60 \text{ minutes}}$$

Next, multiply the fraction by the drip factor (the number of drops contained in 1 ml) to determine the number of drops per minute to be infused. The drip factor varies among I.V. administration sets; follow the manufacturer's guidelines (found on the administration set package) for the drip factor. (See also *Intravenous drip rates.*) Standard administration sets have drip factors of 10, 15, or 20 gtt/ml. A microdrip (minidrip) set has a drip factor of 60 gtt/ml. Which set you use depends on the rate and purpose of the infusion. (See *Determining which type of I.V. tubing to use,* page 118.)

Use the following equation to determine the drip rate of an I.V. solution:

$$\text{drops per minute} = \frac{\text{total milliliters}}{\text{total minutes}} \times \text{drip factor}$$

Note that the equation applies both to large-volume solutions that infuse over many hours and to small-volume solutions that infuse in less than 1 hour.

You can modify the equation by first determining the flow rate (the number of milliliters to be infused over 1 hour). For example, if the patient is to receive 1,000 ml over 8 hours, the fraction would be written as:

$$\text{flow rate} = \frac{1,000 \text{ ml}}{8 \text{ hours}}$$

In this example, the flow rate is 125 ml/hour. You will also use the flow rate when working with I.V. infusion pumps to set the number of milliliters to be delivered in 1 hour (see "Electronic Infusion Devices: Controllers and Pumps," pages 145 to 148). You then divide the flow rate by 60 minutes. This fraction would be written as:

$$\text{rate per minute} = \frac{125 \text{ ml/hour}}{60 \text{ minutes}}$$

INTRAVENOUS DRIP RATES

When calculating the drip rate of I.V. solutions, remember that the number of drops required to deliver 1 ml varies with the type of administration set used and the manufacturer. A standard (macrodrip) set delivers from 10 to 20 gtt/ml. A microdrip set delivers 60 gtt/ml.

To calculate the drip rate, you must know the drip factor for each manufacturer's product. As a quick guide, refer to the chart below.

MANUFACTURER AND DRIP FACTOR (GTT/ML)	DROPS/MINUTE TO INFUSE			
	500 ml/ 24 hr	1,000 ml/ 24 hr	1,000 ml/ 10 hr	1,000 ml/ 8 hr
	21 ml/hr	42 ml/hr	100 ml/hr	125 ml/hr
Abbott (15)	5 gtt	10 gtt	25 gtt	31 gtt
Baxter-Travenol (10)	3 gtt	7 gtt	17 gtt	21 gtt
Cutter (20)	7 gtt	14 gtt	34 gtt	42 gtt
IVAC (20)	7 gtt	14 gtt	34 gtt	42 gtt
McGaw (15)	5 gtt	10 gtt	25 gtt	31 gtt

In this example, the rate is 2.08 ml/minute, which can be rounded to 2.1 ml/minute. The rate per minute is then multiplied by the drip factor (found on the administration tubing set package) to determine the number of drops per minute. If, for example, the Abbott administration set is being used, the drip factor is 15 gtt/ml; thus, the equation would be:

$$\text{drip rate} = 2.1 \text{ ml/minute} \times 15 \text{ gtt/ml}$$

In this example, the drip rate is 31.5 gtt/minute, which can be rounded to 32 gtt/minute.

In practice, you may observe the drip rate for 15 seconds — sufficient time to determine whether the rate needs to be adjusted. To calculate the drip rate for 15 seconds, divide the drip rate per minute by 4. In the example, the equation would be written as:

$$\text{drip rate for 15 seconds} = \frac{32 \text{ gtt/minute}}{4}$$

DETERMINING WHICH TYPE OF I.V. TUBING TO USE

Most health care institutions stock I.V. tubing in several sizes. Microdrip (minidrip) tubing delivers 60 gtt/ml, and "standard" or macrodrip tubing delivers 10, 15, or 20 gtt/ml, depending on the manufacturer.

The rate and purpose of the infusion determine whether microdrip or macrodrip tubing should be used. For example, if a patient is to receive a solution at a rate of 125 ml/hour, macrodrip tubing is preferred. If microdrip tubing were used in this instance, the drip rate would be 125 gtt/minute, which is difficult to assess. Conversely, if a patient is to receive a solution at a rate of 10 ml/hour, microdrip tubing is preferred. If macrodrip tubing with a drip factor of 15 gtt/ml were used, the drip rate would be 3 gtt/minute. Maintaining I.V. patency at this rate is nearly impossible.

A good rule of thumb for selecting I.V. tubing is to use macrodrip tubing for any infusion with a rate of at least 80 ml/hour and microdrip tubing for any infusion with a rate of less than 80 ml/hour. Follow your institution's protocols.

Usually only microdrip tubing is used with pediatric patients to prevent fluid overload (see Chapter 7, Other Considerations).

When I.V. controllers and pumps are used, you would use the tubing specifically manufactured to work with that pump.

In this example, the drip rate is 8 gtt/15 seconds. You would then observe the drip chamber for 15 seconds to ensure that 8 drops are delivered.

You also can use these quicker methods to compute I.V. infusion rates. For example, when using a microdrip set, determine the flow rate for 60 minutes. When you multiply by the drip factor (60 gtt/minute), the fractions cancel each other out: the flow rate equals the drip rate. For example, if the flow rate is 125 ml/60 minutes, the equation would be:

$$125 \text{ gtt/minute (drip rate)} = \frac{125 \text{ ml}}{60 \text{ minutes}} \times \frac{60 \text{ gtt}}{1 \text{ ml}}$$

In this example, the number of drops per minute (125) is the same as the number of milliliters of fluid per hour. Rather than spend time calculating the equation, you can simply use the number assigned to the flow rate as the drip rate.

For I.V. administration sets that deliver 10 gtt/ml, divide the flow rate by 6 to find the drip rate. For sets that deliver 15 gtt/ml, divide the flow rate by 4 to find the drip rate. For sets that deliver 20 gtt/ml, divide the flow rate by 3 to find the drip rate. For example, if the ordered flow rate is 125 ml/hour and you're using a Baxter administration set (drip factor of 10 gtt/ml), the equation would be:

$$\frac{125 \text{ ml}}{6} = 20.8 \text{ gtt/minute}$$

In this example, the drip rate is 20.8 gtt/minute, which can be rounded to 21 gtt/minute. The drip rate obtained is the same whether you use this quick method or one of the longer ones.

Patient situations

1. A physician's order calls for 500 ml of $D_5 0.45NS$ to infuse over 12 hours. You need to determine the drip rate for an administration set that delivers 15 gtt/ml.

- Use this equation:

$$X = \frac{500 \text{ ml}}{12 \text{ hr} \times 60 \text{ minutes}} \times 15 \text{ gtt/ml}$$

- Multiply the number of hours by 60 minutes in the denominator of the fraction:

$$X = \frac{500 \text{ ml}}{720 \text{ minutes}} \times 15 \text{ gtt/ml}$$

- Divide the fraction and solve for X:

$$X = 0.69 \text{ ml/minute} \times 15 \text{ gtt/ml}$$

$$X = 10.35 \text{ gtt/minute}$$

The drip rate is 10.35 gtt/minute, which can be rounded to 10 gtt/minute.

2. A physician's order calls for 1,000 ml of D_5W I.V. over 12 hours. You'll be using a Cutter administration tubing set (drip factor is 20 gtt/ml). What is the flow rate (the amount infused in 1 hour) and the drip rate?

- To calculate the flow rate, set up this proportion and solve for X:

$$\frac{1,000 \text{ ml}}{12 \text{ hour}} = \frac{X \text{ ml}}{1 \text{ hour}}$$

The flow rate is 83.3 ml/hour, which can be rounded to 83 ml/hour.

- To find the drip rate, set up this equation and solve for X:

$$X = \frac{83 \text{ ml}}{60 \text{ minutes}} \times \frac{20 \text{ gtt}}{1 \text{ ml}}$$

The drip rate is 27.6 gtt/minute, which can be rounded to 28 gtt/minute.

3. A physician's order states *Infuse D₅0.45NS at 100 ml/hour.* You are using a McGaw administration tubing set (drip factor is 15 gtt/ml). What is the drip rate for 1 minute? What is the drip rate for 15 seconds?

▪ Using the quick method to calculate the drip rate for 1 minute, you would set up this equation:

$$X = \frac{100 \text{ ml/hour}}{4}$$

$$X = 25 \text{ gtt/minute}$$

▪ To find the drip rate for 15 seconds, use the following equation:

$$X = \frac{25 \text{ gtt/minute}}{4}$$

$$X = 6.25 \text{ or } 6 \text{ gtt/15 seconds}$$

4. A physician's order for a pediatric patient states *Infuse D₅0.25NS at 30 ml/hour.* You are using a microdrip administration tubing set (drip factor is 60 gtt/ml). What is the drip rate?

▪ To find the drip rate, set up the equation as follows:

$$X = \frac{30 \text{ ml}}{60 \text{ minutes}} \times \frac{60 \text{ gtt}}{1 \text{ ml}}$$

$$X = 30 \text{ gtt/minute}$$

You could also use the quick method to find the drip rate, knowing that the numerical value of the drip rate is equal to the numerical value of the flow rate when microdrip tubing is used. In this example, because the flow rate is 30, the drip rate is also 30.

LARGE-VOLUME INFUSIONS

Large-volume infusions are administered for several reasons. Patients who cannot consume enough fluid to maintain normal hydration will receive large-volume infusions to maintain fluid status and prevent dehydration. Such patients include those being prepared for GI surgery, those being maintained NPO for diagnostic testing or because of a GI disorder, and those with dysphagia related to neurologic impairment, age, disease, or trauma.

Dehydrated patients receive large-volume infusions to correct fluid deficits and restore circulatory volume. Infants and elderly patients are at greater risk for dehydration than the general patient population — infants because of their proportionately large body surface areas and elderly patients because of age-related skin and tissue changes, decreases in thermoregulation and awareness of thirst, and use of diuretics to manage cardiovascular disease.

Fluid replacement

If a patient is losing a significant volume of fluid because of drainage (such as gastric fluids draining from a nasogastric tube), the physician may order an I.V. infusion to replace the lost fluid. Usually, the infusion is administered in addition to those fluids intended to maintain normal hydration. In such cases, use two I.V. bottle and tubing sets so that the flow and intake of each solution can be monitored and recorded separately. The condition of the insertion site and the amount of fluid to be infused determine whether both solutions can be infused into the same site simultaneously or whether a second site is necessary. If the patient has multiple-lumen central lines, you can infuse replacement fluids through an unused port. (*Note:* Be especially careful when infusing large volumes of fluid in pediatric or geriatric patients. See Chapter 7, Other Considerations, for more information.)

Fluid replacement is usually based on the amount of fluid lost. When the fluid loss can be measured, 1 ml of I.V. fluid is usually provided for every milliliter of fluid lost. The physician's order or institutional policy should specify when the fluid losses are to be measured and replaced. In an intensive care setting, losses may be measured and replaced hourly. In a general patient care unit, fluid losses may be totaled at the end of a shift, with the next shift then replacing the fluids lost during the previous one.

If the fluid loss cannot be measured (as, for example, in a burn patient), a special formula is used to estimate the loss, and the replacement fluids are specified in the physician's orders.

Patient situation

The physician's order reads *I.V. fluids: D₅0.45NS at 150 ml/hour; replace NG drainage ml/ml with NS with 40 mEq KCl/L.* The patient is on a general patient care floor, where the policy is to replace fluids lost during the previous shift. During the night shift, the patient's nasogastric drainage was 650 ml. You are beginning an 8-hour day shift. What are the infusion rates for the patient's maintenance and replacement fluids if the tubings have a drip factor of 15 gtt/ml?

- To calculate the infusion rate for maintenance fluids ($D_5$0.45NS at 150 ml/hour), set up the equation:

$$X = \frac{150 \text{ ml}}{60 \text{ minutes}} \times \frac{15 \text{ gtt}}{1 \text{ ml}}$$

$$X = 37.5, \text{ or } 38 \text{ gtt/minute}$$

- To calculate the infusion rate for replacement fluids (650 ml NS with 40 mEq KCl to run over 8 hours), first set up the proportion:

$$\frac{650 \text{ ml}}{8 \text{ hours}} = \frac{X \text{ ml}}{1 \text{ hour}}$$

$$X = 81 \text{ ml/hour}$$

- Then calculate the drip rate:

$$X = \frac{81 \text{ ml}}{60 \text{ minutes}} \times \frac{15 \text{ gtt}}{1 \text{ ml}}$$

$$X = 20.2, \text{ or } 20 \text{ gtt/minute}$$

Thus, the maintenance fluids should infuse at 38 gtt/minute and the replacement fluids should infuse at 20 gtt/minute.

Fluid challenge

A physician may wish to evaluate a patient's response to an increased intake of fluids, sometimes referred to as a "fluid challenge." This can be accomplished most quickly by increasing the flow rate of the I.V. infusion for a specified time and then reducing it to a maintenance rate. (*Note:* Use caution when greatly increasing the rate of infusion in pediatric and geriatric patients. See Chapter 7, Other Considerations, for more information.)

Patient situation

The physician's order states *I.V. fluids D_5NS at 200 ml/hour × 2 hours, then D_5NS at 80 ml/hour.* The administration set has a drip factor of 20 gtt/ml. What is the drip rate for the I.V. fluids during the first 2 hours (the fluid challenge)? What is the maintenance drip rate?

- To calculate the drip rate for the first 2 hours, set up the equation:

$$X = \frac{200 \text{ ml}}{60 \text{ minutes}} \times \frac{20 \text{ gtt}}{1 \text{ ml}}$$

$$X = 66.7 \text{ or } 67 \text{ gtt/minute}$$

■ To calculate the maintenance drip rate, set up the equation:

$$X = \frac{80 \text{ ml}}{60 \text{ minutes}} \times \frac{20 \text{ gtt}}{1 \text{ ml}}$$

X = 26.7, or 27 gtt/minute

STANDARD I.V. FLUIDS WITH ADDITIVES

Large-volume infusions with additives are administered to maintain or restore hydration or electrolyte status or to supply additional electrolytes, vitamins, or other nutrients. Common additives include potassium chloride, vitamins B and C, and trace elements.

If the additive is not prepackaged in the solution, either by the manufacturer or by the institution's pharmacy, you must prepare the correct amount and add it to the solution. Then, as with other I.V. solutions, you must calculate the flow rate and the drip rate.

Additives to be included in I.V. fluids are part of the physician's order (for example, D_5W with 20 mEq KCl per liter at 100 ml/hour). This order means that 20 mEq of potassium chloride should be in the liter bottle of dextrose 5% in water and that the flow rate for that solution should be 100 ml/hour.

Sometimes, the order calls for more than one additive to be combined in the solution. Before calculating the correct amounts of each material to inject, check a compatibility chart or consult a pharmacist to ensure that the additives are miscible.

To calculate the correct amount of additive, use the same equations as for any prepared liquid medication. And remember that *any additive-containing I.V. solution must be labeled with the time, name, and amount of medication added.*

Patient situations

1. A patient is to receive 1,000 ml of D_5W with 100 mg of thiamine per liter over 10 hours. The thiamine is available in a prepared syringe of 100 mg/ml. How many milliliters of thiamine must you add to the solution?

■ Using the ratio method, set up the proportion:

100 mg:X ml :: 100 mg:1 ml

■ Solve for X:

$$X \text{ ml} \times 100 \text{ mg} = 100 \text{ mg} \times 1 \text{ ml}$$

$$X = \frac{100 \text{ ml}}{100}$$

$$X = 1 \text{ ml}$$

2. A physician's order states *Infuse D₅0.45NS with 30 mEq KCl per liter at 100 ml/hour.* The potassium chloride is available in vials of 20 mEq/10 ml. How many milliliters of potassium chloride should you add to the solution?

■ Using the fraction method, set up the proportion:

$$\frac{30 \text{ mEq}}{X \text{ ml}} = \frac{20 \text{ mEq}}{10 \text{ ml}}$$

$$X \text{ ml} \times 20 \text{ mEq} = 30 \text{ mEq} \times 10 \text{ ml}$$

$$X = \frac{300 \text{ ml}}{20}$$

$$X = 15 \text{ ml}$$

Another way to solve this problem would be to determine the strength of each milliliter of the potassium chloride solution.

■ Set up the proportion:

$$\frac{X \text{ mEq}}{1 \text{ ml}} = \frac{20 \text{ mEq}}{10 \text{ ml}}$$

■ Solve for X:

$$X \text{ mEq} \times 10 \text{ ml} = 20 \text{ mEq} \times 1 \text{ ml}$$

$$X = 2 \text{ mEq}$$

■ Knowing that you have 2 mEq/ml and that you need 30 mEq, you can use the following proportion:

$$\frac{30 \text{ mEq}}{X \text{ ml}} = \frac{2 \text{ mEq}}{1 \text{ ml}}$$

■ Solve for X:

$$X \text{ ml} \times 2 \text{ mEq} = 30 \text{ mEq} \times 1 \text{ ml}$$

$$X = \frac{30 \text{ ml}}{2}$$

$$X = 15 \text{ ml}$$

Medication additives

Medications added to large-volume I.V. solutions may be ordered in ml/hour, mg/hour, or units/hour. These medications include aminophylline, lidocaine, oxytocin, and dopamine. You must know how to calculate the amount of medication to be given to the patient to ensure that the dosage is within safe and therapeutic limits. You can use either of two methods to do this.

In the one-step method, you determine the amount of medication to give the patient in an hour by multiplying the amount of medication in the I.V. solution by the ordered flow rate and then dividing this number by the number of milliliters of solution in the bottle:

$$\text{dose per hour} = \frac{\text{mg of drug} \times \text{flow rate}}{\text{ml of solution}}$$

The dose per hour is expressed as milligrams or units per hour. The physician can change the dosage by changing the flow rate or by ordering a new solution of different concentration.

The second calculation method involves two steps.

■ First, determine the medication's concentration (the number of milligrams or units per milliliter of solution) by dividing the number of milligrams or units of drug added to the bottle by the number of milliliters of solution:

$$\text{concentration} = \frac{\text{mg of drug}}{\text{ml of solution}}$$

■ Next, calculate the amount of medication the patient should receive in 1 hour by using the following equation:

$$\text{dose per hour} = \text{concentration} \times \text{milliliters}$$

Hint: Although the two-step method may seem more cumbersome, it saves calculation time later if the flow rate is changed. You can simply multiply the new flow rate by the concentration to obtain the new dosage.

■ You can also use fractions as follows:

$$\frac{\text{mg of drug}}{\text{ml of solution}} = \frac{\text{X mg}}{\text{ordered flow rate}}$$

■ Solve for X:

$$\text{X mg} \times \text{ml of solution} = \text{mg of drug} \times \text{ordered flow rate}$$

$$\text{X} = \frac{\text{mg of drug} \times \text{ordered flow rate}}{\text{ml of solution}}$$

■ The hourly medication dosage is simpler to calculate using fractions if you know the solution's concentration. The equation becomes:

$$\frac{\text{mg of drug}}{1 \text{ ml}} = \frac{\text{X mg}}{\text{ordered flow rate}}$$

■ Solve for X:

$$\text{X} = \text{mg/ml} \times \text{ordered flow rate}$$

If the physician's order is written in mg/hour or units/hour, you must determine the flow rate needed. To do this, divide the amount of drug in the solution by the volume of solution and then divide this number by the prescribed hourly dosage. The one-step approach uses the following equation:

$$\text{flow rate} = \text{hourly dose} \div \frac{\text{mg of drug}}{\text{ml of solution}}$$

The flow rate is expressed as milliliters per hour. If the physician changes the patient's dosage, the flow rate of the solution should be changed.

Using the second method, you would determine the solution's concentration and then calculate the flow rate needed to deliver the ordered dose, using the following equation:

$$\text{flow rate} = \frac{\text{hourly dose}}{\text{concentration}}$$

■ You can also use fractions, as follows:

$$\frac{\text{ml of solution}}{\text{mg of drug}} = \frac{\text{X ml/hour}}{\text{hourly dose}}$$

■ Solve for X:

$$\text{X ml/hour} \times \text{mg of drug} = \text{ml of solution} \times \text{hourly dose}$$

$$\text{X} = \frac{\text{ml of solution} \times \text{hourly dose}}{\text{mg of drug}}$$

■ The hourly flow rate is simpler to calculate using fractions if you know the solution's concentration. The equation becomes:

$$\text{X ml/hour (flow rate)} = \frac{\text{mg/hour (hourly dose)}}{\text{mg/ml (concentration)}}$$

Patient situations

1. A physician orders 500 mg of aminophylline in 500 ml of D_5W to infuse at 40 ml/hour. What is the hourly dose of aminophylline?

■ Set up the following proportion:

$$\frac{500 \text{ mg}}{500 \text{ ml}} = \frac{X \text{ mg}}{1 \text{ ml}}$$

■ Solve for X:

$$X \text{ mg} \times 500 \text{ ml} = 1 \text{ ml} \times 500 \text{ mg}$$

$$X = 1 \text{ mg}$$

Thus, the solution's concentration is 1 mg/ml. If the patient is to receive 40 ml/hour, you determine the hourly dosage of aminophylline by using the proportion:

$$\frac{X \text{ mg}}{40 \text{ ml}} = \frac{1 \text{ mg}}{1 \text{ ml}}$$

■ Solve for X:

$$X \text{ mg} \times 1 \text{ ml} = 1 \text{ mg} \times 40 \text{ ml}$$

$$X = 40 \text{ mg}$$

When the flow rate of the solution is 40 ml/hour, the patient will receive 40 mg of aminophylline per hour.

2. A medication order states *20,000 U heparin per 500 ml D_5W; give 1,000 U heparin per hour.* What is the hourly flow rate of the infusion?

■ Set up the following proportion, using the fraction approach:

$$\frac{X \text{ ml}}{1,000 \text{ units}} = \frac{500 \text{ ml}}{20,000 \text{ units}}$$

■ Solve for X:

$$X \text{ ml} \times 20,000 \text{ units} = 1,000 \text{ units} \times 500 \text{ ml}$$

$$X = 25 \text{ ml/hour}$$

To administer 1,000 units of heparin per hour, set the flow rate at 25 ml/hour.

Specialty care units
In specialty units, such as the critical care unit and the labor and delivery unit, you will have to perform calculations for medication additives quickly. Many I.V. drugs — such as the antiarrhythmics lidocaine and bretylol, the vasodilators sodium nitroprusside and nitroglycerin, the adrenergics norepinephrine and dopamine, and the obstetric agent magnesium sulfate — are administered in life-threatening situations. You must prepare the drug for infusion, administer it to the patient, and observe the patient to evaluate the drug's effectiveness.

For example, one or more adrenergic drugs will probably be given to a patient in shock to raise cardiac output quickly. Adrenergic medications, given in 250, 500, or 1,000 ml of I.V. solution, are usually ordered in micrograms per minute or micrograms per kilogram per minute. They must be given via infusion pumps, and the flow rate is adjusted, or titrated, to restore and maintain normal blood pressure. If more than one adrenergic drug is ordered, each must be diluted and infused in a separate solution.

When administering these types of medications, you must calculate the drug's concentration in the I.V. solution and the flow rate required to deliver the desired dose. You also may have to calculate the number of micrograms needed, based on the patient's weight in kilograms.

To calculate the drug's concentration, use the following equation:

$$\text{concentration (in mg/ml)} = \frac{\text{mg of medication}}{\text{ml of fluid}}$$

(To convert the concentration from milligrams to micrograms, multiply by 1,000.)

You can use either of two methods to calculate the I.V. flow rate. In one method, you would determine the flow rate per minute, using the following proportion:

$$\frac{\text{dose/minute}}{\text{X ml/minute}} = \frac{\text{concentration of solution}}{\text{1 ml of fluid}}$$

In the other method, you would first multiply the ordered dose, given in micrograms per minute, by 60 minutes to determine the hourly dose. Next, use the following proportion to compute the hourly flow rate:

$$\frac{\text{hourly dose}}{\text{X ml}} = \frac{\text{concentration of solution}}{\text{1 ml of fluid}}$$

To ensure that the drug is being given in the safe and therapeutic range, you can determine the amount of medication given (in mg/kg/minute) and compare it to information shown in a drug reference. The calculation involves several steps.

■ First, determine the solution's concentration, as explained previously. Then, determine the amount of medication being given to the patient by multiplying the flow rate by the concentration:

medication received (mg/hour) = flow rate × concentration

▪ Next, to calculate the dose being received by the patient each minute, divide the hourly amount by 60 minutes:

$$\text{mg/minute} = \frac{\text{mg/hour}}{60 \text{ minutes}}$$

▪ Then, divide the amount of medication received by the patient each minute by the patient's weight:

$$\text{mg/kg/minute} = \frac{\text{mg/minute}}{\text{weight (kg)}}$$

Now you can compare this amount to the dosage information in a drug reference.

At times, the pharmacy may prepare the solution and label it as follows: 500 ml D₅W, nitroglycerin, 4:1. You can calculate the solution's concentration from this information. The first number in the ratio refers to the amount of medication (in milligrams); the second number, to the amount of diluent (in milliliters). In the example, 4 mg of nitroglycerin are diluted in 1 ml of D₅W. Thus, the concentration is 4 mg/ml.

Patient situations: Critical care

1. A physician's order for a patient in shock states *4 mg norepinephrine per 250 ml D₅W, administer at 12 mcg/minute.* What is the rate of infusion in milliliters per minute? In milliliters per hour?

▪ To find the solution's strength, use the following proportion:

$$\frac{\text{X mg}}{1 \text{ ml}} = \frac{4 \text{ mg}}{250 \text{ ml}}$$

▪ Solve for X:

$$\text{X mg} \times 250 \text{ ml} = 1 \text{ ml} \times 4 \text{ mg}$$

$$\text{X} = \frac{4 \text{ mg}}{250}$$

$$\text{X} = 0.016 \text{ mg}$$

$$\text{X} = 16 \text{ mcg}$$

▪ To calculate the flow rate needed to deliver the ordered dose of 12 mcg/minute, use the following proportion:

$$\frac{12 \text{ mcg/minute}}{\text{X ml}} = \frac{16 \text{ mcg}}{1 \text{ ml}}$$

■ Solve for X:

$$X \text{ ml} \times 16 \text{ mcg} = 12 \text{ mcg/minute} \times 1 \text{ ml}$$

$$X = \frac{12 \text{ ml/minute}}{16}$$

$$X = 0.75 \text{ ml/minute}$$

The patient should receive 0.75 ml/minute.

■ Since infusion pumps are used when administering norepinephrine, you should also compute the hourly rate:

$$\frac{X \text{ ml}}{60 \text{ minutes}} = \frac{0.75 \text{ ml}}{1 \text{ minute}}$$

■ Solve for X:

$$X \text{ ml} \times 1 \text{ minute} = 60 \text{ minutes} \times 0.75 \text{ ml}$$

$$X = 45 \text{ ml}$$

Set the infusion pump to deliver 45 ml/hour.

2. A patient is to receive an I.V. infusion of procainamide at 3 mg/minute. The pharmacist labels the solution *250 ml D₅W, procainamide, 4:1.* How many milliliters of solution should the patient receive each minute?

■ First, determine the solution's concentration. Since the 4 in the ratio is the amount of procainamide and the 1 is the amount of D_5W in which the procainamide is diluted, the solution's concentration is 4 mg/ml.

■ Next, calculate the flow rate needed to deliver the ordered dose of 3 mg/minute:

$$\frac{3 \text{ mg/minute}}{X \text{ ml}} = \frac{4 \text{ mg}}{1 \text{ ml}}$$

■ Solve for X:

$$X \text{ ml} \times 4 \text{ mg} = 3 \text{ mg/minute} \times 1 \text{ ml}$$

$$X = \frac{3 \text{ ml/minute}}{4}$$

The patient should receive 0.75 ml/minute. (*Note:* Because an infusion pump will be used, you should also compute the hourly rate, as in Patient Situation 1 above.)

3. A physician's order states *2 amp dopamine in 500 ml D₅W; infuse at 12 ml/hour.* Each ampule contains 200 mg. If the patient weighs

150 pounds, how much medication (in mcg/kg/minute) will he receive?

■ Because each ampule contains 200 mg of dopamine, a total of 400 mg of dopamine will be added to the D_5W (200 mg/amp × 2 amp = 400 mg). With this information, you can determine the solution's concentration by using the proportion:

$$\frac{X \text{ mg}}{1 \text{ ml}} = \frac{400 \text{ mg}}{500 \text{ ml}}$$

$$X \text{ mg} \times 500 \text{ ml} = 1 \text{ ml} \times 400 \text{ mg}$$

$$X = \frac{400 \text{ mg}}{500}$$

$$X = 0.8 \text{ mg or } 800 \text{ mcg}$$

■ The concentration is 800 mcg/ml. Next, determine the amount of medication the patient receives each hour by using the equation:

$$X = 12 \text{ ml/hour} \times 800 \text{ mcg/ml}$$

$$X = 9{,}600 \text{ mcg/hour}$$

■ The patient is receiving 9,600 mcg/hour. Next, determine the dose per minute by dividing the hourly amount by 60 minutes:

$$X = \frac{9{,}600 \text{ mcg}}{60 \text{ minutes}}$$

$$X = 160 \text{ mcg/minute}$$

■ The patient is receiving 160 mcg/minute. Next, convert the patient's weight from pounds to kilograms:

$$\frac{X \text{ kg}}{150 \text{ lb}} = \frac{1 \text{ kg}}{2.2 \text{ lb}}$$

$$X = \frac{150 \text{ kg}}{2.2}$$

$$X = 68.2 \text{ kg}$$

■ The patient weighs 68.2 kg. Now, you can calculate the amount of medication received each minute per kilogram of body weight by using the equation:

$$X = \frac{160 \text{ mcg/minute}}{68.2 \text{ kg}}$$

$$X = 2.3 \text{ mcg/kg/minute}$$

The patient is receiving 2.3 mcg/kg/minute.

4. A physician's order states *2 amp dopamine in 500 ml D₅W; infuse at 300 mcg/minute.* If each ampule contains 200 mg, how many milliliters per hour should the patient receive?

▪ As in Patient Situation 3, you would determine that the solution contains 400 mg of dopamine and that the concentration is 800 mcg/ml. To calculate the hourly amount of medication needed, multiply 300 mcg/minute by 60 minutes (18,000 mcg/hour). Next, to determine the amount of solution needed to administer this dose, set up the proportion:

$$\frac{\text{X ml}}{18,000 \text{ mcg/hour}} = \frac{1 \text{ ml}}{800 \text{ mcg}}$$

$$X = \frac{18,000 \text{ ml}}{800 \text{ hour}}$$

$$X = 22.5 \text{ or } 23 \text{ ml/hour}$$

Set the infusion pump to deliver 23 ml/hour.

5. A physician's order states *2 amp dopamine in 500 ml D₅W; administer at 5 mcg/kg/minute.* If each ampule contains 200 mg and the patient weighs 150 pounds, how many milliliters should he receive each hour?

▪ As in Patient Situation 3, you would first determine that the solution's concentration is 800 mcg/ml and that the patient weighs 68.2 kg. If the patient is to receive 5 mcg/kg/minute, multiply 68.2 by 5 (341 mcg/minute). To calculate the hourly dose, multiply 341 mcg/minute by 60 minutes (20,460 mcg/hour).

▪ Finally, to determine the amount of solution needed to administer this dose, use the proportion:

$$\frac{\text{X ml}}{20,460 \text{ mcg/hour}} = \frac{1 \text{ ml}}{800 \text{ mcg}}$$

▪ Solve for X:

$$\text{X ml} \times 800 \text{ mcg} = 20,460 \text{ mcg/hour} \times 1 \text{ ml}$$

$$X = \frac{20,460 \text{ ml}}{800 \text{ hour}}$$

$$X = 25.5 \text{ or } 26 \text{ ml/hour}$$

Set the infusion pump to deliver 26 ml/hour.

6. A patient has been resuscitated after cardiac arrest. The physician orders 1 G of lidocaine added to 250 ml of D₅W, to be infused at 4 mg/minute. What is the hourly infusion rate?

- First, calculate the solution's concentration, using the proportion:

$$\frac{X \text{ mg}}{1 \text{ ml}} = \frac{1,000 \text{ mg}}{250 \text{ ml}}$$

- Solve for X:

$$X \text{ mg} \times 250 \text{ ml} = 1 \text{ ml} \times 1,000 \text{ mg}$$

$$X = \frac{1,000 \text{ mg}}{250}$$

$$X = 4 \text{ mg}$$

- The concentration is 4 mg/ml. Now compute the hourly dose by multiplying the dose per minute by 60 minutes:

$$4 \text{ mg/minute} \times 60 \text{ minutes/hour} = 240 \text{ mg/hour}$$

- The patient should receive 240 mg/hour. To determine the amount of lidocaine solution needed to administer the 240 mg, set up the following proportion:

$$\frac{X \text{ ml}}{240 \text{ mg}} = \frac{1 \text{ ml}}{4 \text{ mg}}$$

- Solve for X:

$$X \text{ ml} \times 4 \text{ mg} = 240 \text{ mg} \times 1 \text{ ml}$$

$$X = \frac{240 \text{ ml}}{40}$$

$$X = 60 \text{ ml}$$

The infusion rate should be 60 ml/hour.

Patient situations: Obstetrics

1. A physician orders oxytocin, as follows, to stimulate labor: *1 ml Pitocin (10 U) in 1 L NSS; infuse at 1 mU/minute for 20 minutes, then increase flow rate to 2 mU/minute.* Pitocin must be given via an I.V. pump. What is the concentration of the solution? What is the flow rate needed to deliver 1 milliunit/minute for 20 minutes? What is the flow rate needed to deliver 2 milliunits/minute thereafter?

- You can determine the solution's concentration by using the following proportion:

$$\frac{10 \text{ units}}{1,000 \text{ ml}} = \frac{X \text{ unit}}{1 \text{ ml}}$$

■ Solve for X:

$$X \text{ units} \times 1,000 \text{ ml} = 10 \text{ units} \times 1 \text{ ml}$$

$$X = \frac{10 \text{ units}}{1,000}$$

$$X = 0.01 \text{ unit}$$

This can be written in milliunits (mU, thousandths of a unit). In this case, .01 unit = 10 milliunits, so the concentration is 10 milliunits/ml.

■ If the patient is to receive 1 milliunit/minute for 20 minutes, then he should receive a total of 20 milliunits. To calculate the flow rate needed to provide that dosage, use the following proportion:

$$\frac{10 \text{ milliunits}}{1 \text{ ml}} = \frac{20 \text{ milliunits}}{X \text{ ml}}$$

■ Solve for X:

$$X \text{ ml} \times 10 \text{ milliunits} = 1 \text{ ml} \times 20 \text{ milliunits}$$

$$X = \frac{20 \text{ ml}}{10}$$

$$X = 2 \text{ ml}$$

The flow rate would be 2 ml/20 minutes. Because an I.V. pump must be used to deliver this medication, you must compute the hourly flow rate. Multiplying the 20-minute rate by 3, you would determine that you must set the pump to deliver 6 ml/hour.

■ Remember, however, that you must change this rate after 20 minutes. You also must calculate the flow rate to be used after the first 20 minutes to provide 2 milliunits/minute (or 120 milliunits/hour). Having calculated the solution's concentration as 10 milliunits/ml, you would use the following proportion:

$$\frac{10 \text{ milliunits}}{1 \text{ ml}} = \frac{120 \text{ milliunits}}{X \text{ ml}}$$

■ Solve for X:

$$X \text{ ml} \times 10 \text{ milliunits} = 1 \text{ ml} \times 120 \text{ milliunits}$$

$$X = \frac{120 \text{ ml}}{10}$$

$$X = 12 \text{ ml}$$

Thus, after 20 minutes, you should reset the pump to deliver 12 ml/hour.

Here's a simpler approach to the last part of this situation: Since the dose has been doubled (from 1 to 2 milliunits/minute), the flow rate should also be doubled (from 6 to 12 ml/hour).

2. A physician orders magnesium sulfate, 4 G in 250 ml D_5W, to be infused at 1 G/hour. What is the flow rate (ml/hour)?

One approach is to use the following proportion:

$$\frac{4\ G}{250\ ml} = \frac{1\ G}{X\ ml}$$

■ Solve for X:

$$X\ ml \times 4\ G = 250\ ml \times 1\ G$$

$$X = \frac{250\ ml}{4}$$

$$X = 62.5\ or\ 63\ ml$$

The magnesium sulfate solution should be infused at 63 ml/hour.

■ Another approach is to calculate the strength of the solution:

$$\frac{4\ G}{250\ ml} = \frac{X\ G}{1\ ml}$$

■ Solve for X:

$$X\ G \times 250\ ml = 4\ G \times 1\ ml$$

$$X = \frac{4\ G}{250}$$

$$X = 0.016\ G$$

■ Next, calculate the flow rate as follows:

$$\frac{X\ ml}{1\ G} = \frac{1\ ml}{0.016\ G}$$

■ Solve for X:

$$X\ ml \times 0.016\ G = 1\ ml \times 1\ G$$

$$X = \frac{1\ ml}{0.016}$$

$$X = 62.5\ or\ 63\ ml$$

Note that the same flow rate is obtained using either method.

SMALL-VOLUME INFUSIONS

Some medications are added to a small volume of I.V. solution and the resultant solution is administered in less than 1 hour. These small-volume infusions are called "piggybacks" because they are connected (piggybacked) to an existing I.V. line or venous access device, such as a heparin lock or central line (see "Venous access devices," pages 148 to 150).

If your institution's pharmacy does not add the medication to the infusion, you'll have to prepare the medication, using the calculations discussed earlier in this chapter.

Antibiotics are the piggybacks administered most frequently. Because some antibiotics lose their potency quickly, check the label to ensure that the medication is prepared and administered within the required time. For example, an ampicillin piggyback should be administered within 1 hour of the reconstitution of the ampicillin powder. For this reason, any I.V. solution that contains additives should be labeled with the time, name of medication, and amount of medication added. Also make sure the I.V. solution is compatible with the medication. For instance, although many piggybacks can be added to D_5W, phenytoin can be administered only in normal (0.9%) saline solution.

The equipment used to administer piggybacks also varies among institutions and may include the following:

■ small-volume (50 ml to 250 ml) solution bottle or bag, to which medication is added

■ small-volume (50 ml to 250 ml) solution bag with a special port permitting a medication vial to be attached and contents of the medication vial mixed with the solution

■ syringe of appropriately concentrated medication and a micro-infuser line on an electronic regulation device

■ I.V. solution bottle or bag (250 ml to 500 ml) attached to a 100-ml rigid plastic cylinder. The solution flows from the bottle or bag into the plastic cylinder, and the medication is added to the plastic cylinder to permit mixing with the solution.

The prepared small-volume infusion may be attached to an existing I.V. line (either with a Y-type attachment port or through tubing and needle to a rubber port on the I.V. line) or to a peripheral or central venous access device. Before attaching a piggyback to an existing I.V. line, consult a compatibility chart or check with the pharmacy to make sure the two solutions are compatible, especially if both contain additives.

Infusion time varies, depending on the medication, the volume of fluid to be infused, and institutional policies and procedures. Usually, you'll administer volumes under 100 ml in 1 hour or less and volumes under 50 ml in ½ hour or less.

Patient situations

1. A patient is to receive 50 ml of an I.V. penicillin solution over 30 minutes. The set has a drip factor of 15 gtt/ml. What is the drip rate?

■ Set up the equation and solve for X:

$$X = \frac{50 \text{ ml}}{30 \text{ minutes}} \times 15 \text{ gtt/ml}$$

$$X = \frac{750 \text{ gtt}}{30 \text{ minutes}}$$

$$X = 25 \text{ gtt/minute}$$

2. A patient is to receive 100 ml of an I.V. gentamicin solution over 1 hour. The set has a drip factor of 20 gtt/ml. What is the drip rate?

■ Set up the equation and solve for X:

$$X = \frac{100 \text{ ml}}{60 \text{ minutes}} \times 20 \text{ gtt/ml}$$

$$X = \frac{2,000 \text{ gtt}}{60 \text{ minutes}}$$

$$X = 33.3 \text{ or } 33 \text{ gtt/minute}$$

3. A patient is to receive 30 ml of an I.V. dexamethasone solution over 10 minutes. The set has a drip factor of 10 gtt/ml. What is the drip rate?

■ Set up the equation and solve for X:

$$X = \frac{30 \text{ ml}}{10 \text{ minutes}} \times 10 \text{ gtt/ml}$$

$$X = \frac{300 \text{ gtt}}{10 \text{ minutes}}$$

$$X = 30 \text{ gtt/minute}$$

Hint: The institution's policy or the physician's order may provide for a range of time (for instance, 20 to 40 minutes) over which the solution must be infused. Unless contraindicated, you can use any infusion time within the range that will simplify your calculations. For example:

You may choose to infuse a 50-ml piggyback over 25 minutes (selected from an ordered range of 15 to 30 minutes) because this simplifies the equation:

$$X = \frac{2\,50\text{ ml}}{25\text{ minutes}} \times \text{drip factor (gtt/ml)}$$

Suppose the drip factor is 15 gtt/ml. Infusing the piggyback over 30 minutes simplifies the equation:

$$X = \frac{50\text{ ml}}{2\,30\text{ minutes}} \times 15\text{ gtt/ml}$$

OTHER INFUSIONS

Besides medications, other products may be administered directly into the patient's bloodstream. These include total parenteral nutrition (TPN) and blood and blood products. Additionally, some medications are infused with electronic infusion devices — such as patient-controlled analgesia (PCA) systems and infusion pumps — that require special calculations.

Total parenteral nutrition

A patient receives parenteral nutrition when nutrient needs cannot be met enterally because of elevated requirements or impaired digestion or absorption in the GI tract. TPN — also called central parenteral nutrition (CPN) or intravenous hyperalimentation (IVH or HAL) — can be administered centrally via the superior vena cava, inferior vena cava, or right atrium, or peripherally via the veins of the arms, legs, or scalp. Most institutions have a written protocol regarding insertion site and recommended solutions.

Parenteral nutrition is available in commercially prepared products or individually formulated solutions from the pharmacy. Because of the potential for patient infection, the solutions are prepared under sterile and carefully monitored conditions. Nurses rarely are responsible for preparing these solutions on the patient unit.

Parenteral nutrition solutions contain a 10% or greater dextrose concentration. Amino acids are provided to maintain or restore nitrogen balance, and vitamins, electrolytes, and trace minerals are added to meet individual needs. Lipids also are provided but are given separately to prevent their destruction by the other nutrients. (*Note:* Because additives increase a solution's total volume, they affect intake measurements. For example, if you're assessing the amount of fluid remaining in the patient's TPN bottle and you find 20 to 50 ml more than you expected, determine whether the volume of additives explains the discrepancy.)

Initially, TPN is infused at a slow rate, which is gradually increased to a maintenance level. Similarly, the rate is gradually decreased before discontinuing TPN. Most TPN solutions are administered via infusion pump.

Patient situations

1. A patient with ileitis is receiving TPN. The physician's order states *500 ml 7.5% Aminosyn + 500 ml 20% dextrose I.V. to infuse over 10 hours.* The solution was hung at 10 p.m. How many milliliters remain in the bottle at 3 a.m.?

■ First, calculate the hourly flow rate, as follows:

$$\frac{1,000 \text{ ml}}{10 \text{ hours}} = \frac{X \text{ ml}}{1 \text{ hour}}$$

$$X = 100 \text{ ml/hour}$$

■ If an I.V. pump is being used, the hourly rate should be set at 100 ml/hour. (If not, then you must calculate the drip rate.) Next, calculate the amount of solution that should have been administered by 3 a.m. Since the solution has been infusing for 5 hours at 100 ml/hour, the equation would be:

$$X = 5 \text{ hours} \times 100 \text{ ml/hour}$$

$$X = 500 \text{ ml}$$

■ Next, calculate the amount of fluid remaining by subtracting the amount of fluid infused from the amount of solution hung:

$$
\begin{array}{r}
1,000 \text{ ml} \\
- \quad 500 \text{ ml} \\
\hline
500 \text{ ml}
\end{array}
$$

Thus, 500 ml should remain in the bottle at 3 a.m. (*Note:* See *Time-taping an I.V. solution,* page 140, for more information on monitoring infusion rates.)

TIME-TAPING AN I.V. SOLUTION

To ensure that you administer an I.V. solution at the prescribed rate and to facilitate your recording of intake fluids, you can time-tape the bag. Some institutions require you to do this and may provide labels for this purpose.

To time-tape an I.V. bag, place a piece of adhesive tape from the top to the bottom of the bag, next to the markings that indicate fluid level (see the illustration below, which shows a bag time-taped for a rate of 100 ml/hour). Next to the "0" marking, record the time that you hang the bag. Then, knowing the hourly rate, mark each hour on the tape next to the corresponding fluid marking. At the bottom of the tape, mark the time at which the solution will be completely infused.

Note: Don't write directly on I.V. bags with felt-tip markers because the ink may seep into the I.V. fluid.

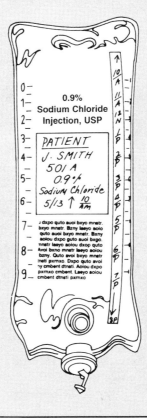

2. A burn patient is receiving TPN. The physician's order states *500 ml 8.5% Aminosyn + 500 ml 20% dextrose I.V. with 1 ampule trace elements + 1 ampule multivitamins + 1 ampule MgSO₄ to infuse over 8 hours.* The solution was hung at 8 a.m. How many milliliters remain in the bottle at 2 p.m.?

■ First, calculate the hourly flow rate, as follows:

$$X = \frac{1{,}000 \text{ ml}}{8 \text{ hours}}$$

$$X = 125 \text{ ml/hour}$$

■ If an I.V. pump is being used, the hourly rate should be set at 125 ml/hour. (If not, then you must calculate the drip rate.) Next, calculate the amount of solution that should have been administered by 2 p.m. Because the solution has been infusing for 6 hours at 125 ml/hour, the equation would be:

$$X = 6 \text{ hours} \times 125 \text{ ml/hour}$$

$$X = 750 \text{ ml}$$

■ Next, calculate the amount of fluid remaining by subtracting the amount of fluid infused from the amount of solution hung:

$$\begin{array}{r} 1{,}000 \text{ ml} \\ - \quad 750 \text{ ml} \\ \hline 250 \text{ ml} \end{array}$$

Thus, 250 ml should remain in the bottle at 2 p.m. You may note, however, that 275 ml remain. The ampules of additives (trace elements, multivitamins, and MgSO₄) may explain the discrepancy.

3. The physician's orders for a comatose patient state *500 ml of 20% Liposyn over 4 hours q. Mon., Wed., and Fri.* What is the hourly flow rate? If the infusion is started at 10 a.m., how much of the solution should be infused by 12:30 p.m.?

■ To calculate the hourly flow rate, use the following equation and solve for X:

$$X = \frac{500 \text{ ml}}{4 \text{ hours}}$$

$$X = 125 \text{ ml/hour}$$

■ To calculate the amount of solution that should be infused by 12:30 p.m. (2.5 hours after the infusion was begun), use the proportion:

$$\frac{X \text{ ml}}{2.5 \text{ hours}} = \frac{125 \text{ ml}}{1 \text{ hour}}$$

■ Solve for X:

$$X = 2.5 \times 125 \text{ ml}$$
$$X = 312.5 \text{ or } 313 \text{ ml}$$

About 313 ml of 20% Liposyn should be infused by 12:30 p.m.

Blood and blood products

The transfusion of blood and blood products requires special administration sets that contain filters to remove agglutinated cells. The drip factor for blood administration sets is usually 10 to 15 gtt/ml, and an 18G or larger needle is used for the I.V. insertion. These factors help prevent cell damage and ensure an adequate flow rate.

Most institutions have specific protocols for the transfusion of blood and blood products. For example, a unit (about 250 to 275 ml) of whole blood or packed red blood cells (RBCs) should infuse for no more than 4 hours because significant deterioration and bacterial contamination of the blood may occur after this time. Many institutions suggest that such a transfusion should be completed in about 2 hours. Note, however, that this rate may be too fast for pediatric and geriatric patients (see Chapter 7, Other Considerations).

In addition, you must take special precautions when transfusing blood products, such as platelets, cryoprecipitate, and granulocytes. Consult your institution's procedure manual to determine the type of tubing to use and the suggested rate and duration of the transfusion.

Patient situation

The physician's order states *Transfuse 1 unit packed RBCs as soon as available from blood bank.* The patient is a young adult with no known cardiac impairment. The transfusion set has a drip factor of 10 gtt/ml. What is the transfusion rate? What is the drip rate?

■ To calculate the transfusion rate, set up the proportion:

$$\frac{250 \text{ ml}}{2 \text{ hours}} = \frac{X \text{ ml}}{1 \text{ hour}}$$
$$X = 125 \text{ ml/hour}$$

■ To calculate the drip rate, set up the equation:

$$X = \frac{125 \text{ ml}}{60 \text{ minutes}} \times 10 \text{ gtt/ml}$$

$$X = 20.8 \text{ or } 21 \text{ gtt/minute}$$

Note: Don't add blood or blood products to an I.V. line that contains dextrose or calcium solutions. Dextrose solutions cause cell hemolysis; calcium solutions, such as lactated Ringer's solution, can cause clotting. Normal saline solution is compatible with blood and blood products.

Patient-controlled analgesia (PCA)

PCA devices are specially designed I.V. infusion pumps that allow patients to self-administer analgesic medication (see photograph on page 144). The computerized pump, which is attached to the patient's I.V. line, is programmed by the nurse (or, in some situations, by the patient or caregiver) to deliver a precise dose of pain medication, usually morphine, at a steady rate (basal dose) or when the patient pushes the control button.

PCA devices provide consistent blood concentrations of pain medication and are considered superior to the traditional pain-relief approach, in which the nurse administers analgesic medication every few hours, usually by the intramuscular route. The traditional approach produces vacillating blood levels of analgesic medication, resulting in periods of heavy sedation alternating with periods of increasing pain. An added benefit of PCA devices is that patients tend to take less medication than they would with the more traditional approach. PCA also is considered superior to continuous I.V. infusion of analgesic medication because the patient gains a measure of pain control.

Several safety features are built into PCA devices. For example, the medication dose and administration frequency are programmed into the machine. If the patient pushes the button more frequently, the machine ignores the requests, thus preventing overdose. Furthermore, the machine records both filled and unfilled requests for medication; the PCA's log shows the number of attempts and the number of times the patient actually received the medication. Thus, you will know if your patient is continually requesting more medication, and you can evaluate his need for it.

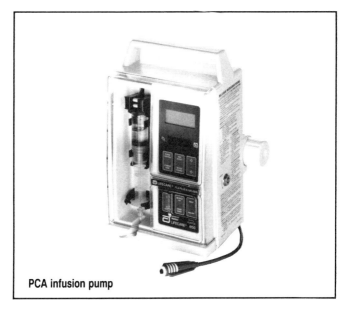

PCA infusion pump

PCA devices require use of an access code or key before entering drug dose and frequency information into the system. This prevents accidental resetting or tampering with the device by unauthorized persons. In addition, some machines record unauthorized entries.

When caring for a patient receiving PCA, follow these guidelines:

■ Draw up the correct amount and concentration of medication, and insert it into the PCA device.

■ Program the device according to the manufacturer's directions (an average setting is 1 mg of morphine every 6 minutes or longer).

■ Read and interpret the PCA log, and record the information on the patient's medication record.

When you interpret the PCA log, note the strength (the number of milligrams per milliliter) of the medication solution in the PCA syringe. You need this information to calculate the dose received by the patient. (The nurse who fills the syringe should record the solution's strength.) Note the basal dose, if the patient is receiving one, and the number of times the patient received medication during the time being assessed (usually every 4 hours). If you multiply the number of injections received by the volume of each injection, you can determine the amount of solution received by the patient. Then multiply this amount by the strength of the solution, as shown in this equation:

fluid volume × solution strength = total medication received

Record the result (the milligrams of drug received) in the patient's medication record.

Most institutions require the nurse who fills the syringe to record the amount of fluid and the amount of medication in the syringe. Each nurse who checks the PCA log also records this information. The data enable you to double-check the accuracy of your calculations.

Patient situation

When reading a patient's PCA log, you note that he received a basal dose of 1 mg of morphine per hour and that he requested and received four injections of 2 ml each, over 4 hours. The medication record indicates that 1 ml of solution contains 1 mg of morphine. The syringe was filled with 30 ml of fluid 4 hours ago; 18 ml remain. The nurse who filled the syringe recorded that the syringe contained 30 mg of morphine. How much medication did the patient receive?

■ First, note the strength of the solution (1 mg/ml). Next, calculate the amount of fluid received in the basal dose:

4 hours × 1 ml/hour = 4 ml

■ Next, calculate the amount of additional fluid requested and received by the patient:

4 injections × 2 ml = 8 ml

■ Then, calculate to total amount of fluid received by adding the basal dose and requested dose amounts:

4 ml + 8 ml = 12 ml

■ To determine the amount of morphine the patient received, use the equation:

12 ml × 1 mg/ml = 12 mg

To double-check, subtract the amount of fluid received (12 ml) from the amount in the syringe at the last log check (30 ml). The result should equal the amount remaining in the machine (18 ml). You can also double-check your calculations based on the actual medication dosage. The syringe originally contained 30 mg of morphine with a strength of 1 mg/ml. Since you calculated that the patient received 12 mg, then 18 mg (18 ml) should remain.

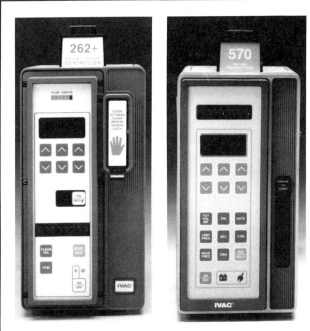

Electronic volumetric controller and electronic infusion pump

Electronic infusion devices: Controllers and pumps

Electronic infusion devices, such as infusion controllers and infusion pumps, facilitate I.V. administration (see photographs above). Infusion controllers regulate the rate of gravity-fed infusions by electronically counting or measuring drops or by determining the rate based on volume. Infusion pumps administer fluid under positive pressure and may be calibrated by drip rate or volume. Some new devices have variable pressure limits that prevent them from pumping fluids into infiltrated sites.

These devices permit you to control the infusion rate by setting the volume or drip rate, shorten the time needed to calibrate an infusion rate, require less maintenance, and provide greater accuracy than the standard methods that drip fluid by gravity. Additionally, some devices keep track of the amount of fluid that has been infused, which helps you maintain accurate intake and output records. Many devices include alarms that signal when the fluid container is empty or when a mechanical problem occurs.

The nurse sets the infuser to deliver a constant amount of solution per minute or hour. Since each infusion device has its own operating instructions, follow the manufacturer's guidelines to ensure adequate functioning of the pump.

When working with a controller or pump, you must program it based on calculation of the infusion rate. An electronic infusion device does not eliminate the need for careful calculations and attention to infusion rates over time.

To determine the pump settings, consider the amount of fluid to be given and the time over which it must be infused. With most devices, you must program the amount of fluid to be infused and the hourly flow rate. With others, you must program the flow rate per minute or the drip rate. For example, suppose that a patient is to receive 1,000 ml of fluid over 8 hours. You would enter 1,000 ml into the infuser's program as the amount of fluid to be infused. Next, you would calculate the hourly flow rate:

$$X = \frac{1,000 \text{ ml}}{8 \text{ hours}}$$

$$X = 125 \text{ ml/hour}$$

If you're using a device that requires you to calculate the flow rate per minute, use the equation:

$$X = \frac{125 \text{ ml}}{60 \text{ minutes}}$$

$$X = 2.1 \text{ ml/minute}$$

Finally, to calculate the drip rate, use the equation:

$$X = 2.1 \text{ ml/minute} \times 15 \text{ gtt/ml (drip factor)}$$

$$X = 31.5 \text{ or } 32 \text{ gtt/minute}$$

Hint: You may set the total volume to be infused at slightly less than the amount ordered. For example, if 1 L of fluid is ordered and hung, set the infuser to 950 ml. Then, when the preset volume is reached (in this case, 950 ml) and the infuser alarm reminds you to hang the next bottle, you'll have extra time to do so. You can reset the infuser for the remaining amount of fluid (50 ml) and, while that is infusing, prepare the next I.V. bottle.

Infusion devices are especially helpful when the infusion contains medication additives. A correctly programmed infuser provides greater assurance that the patient will receive the ordered rate and volume of medication. For example, if a patient with respiratory difficulty is receiving an aminophylline drip (500 mg/250 ml at 25 ml/hour), you would set the hourly rate at 25 ml and the total volume at 250 ml. The infusion pump prevents the common alterations in flow related to patient position (or warns you, via the alarm system, should these changes occur) and ensures a more even administration and drug blood level.

Patient situation

The physician's order states *Infuse 1,000 ml D$_5$0.45NS over 10 hours.* The patient has an I.V. controller that you must set with information about the volume of fluid to be infused and the flow rate in drops per minute. How would you proceed?

■ First, determine the hourly flow rate using this equation:

$$X = \frac{1,000 \text{ ml}}{10 \text{ hours}}$$

$$X = 100 \text{ ml/hour}$$

■ Next, determine the flow rate per minute using this equation:

$$X = \frac{100 \text{ ml}}{60 \text{ minutes}}$$

$$X = 1.7 \text{ ml/minute}$$

■ Finally, calculate the drip rate using this equation:

$$X = 1.7 \text{ ml/minute} \times 10 \text{ gtt/ml (drip factor)}$$

$$X = 17 \text{ gtt/minute}$$

Thus, you would set the volume of fluid to be infused at 1,000 ml and the drip rate at 17 gtt/minute.

Venous access devices

Venous access devices permit continuous or intermittent infusions of solutions and rapid administration of emergency medications. Venous access devices inserted into a peripheral vein for intermittent infusion are called heparin locks. The hub of the cannula is occluded with a cap or adapter rather than being attached to I.V. tubing. Normal saline solution or heparin is administered intermittently to maintain patency of the I.V. line.

Venous access devices are inserted into central veins when peripheral venous access is difficult or when the patient requires frequent venous access over an extended period, such as during a chemotherapy regimen or when receiving TPN. Among these venous access devices are single- and multiple-lumen central lines, Hickman and Groshong catheters, and implantable infusion devices (shown at right).

IMPLANTABLE INFUSION DEVICES

An implantable infusion device, such as the one illustrated here, can be inserted into a central vein when access to a peripheral vein is difficult or when the patient requires frequent venous access over an extended time. Such devices must be flushed periodically to maintain patency.

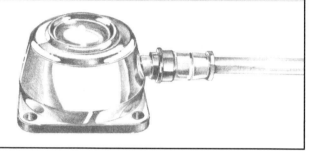

Venous access devices for intermittent infusions must be "flushed" to maintain patency. The frequency depends, in part, on the type of device used and its purpose. For example, a peripheral venous access device being used for potential emergency medication may be flushed once per shift to ensure patency. One being used for intermittent infusions of small-volume solutions containing antibiotics may be flushed with saline before and after each infusion. A central venous access device may be flushed with saline before each intermittent infusion and with saline and heparin after the infusion. If the port on a central venous access device is not being used, it may be flushed with saline or heparin once per shift, or according to institution policy, to ensure patency. An implanted venous access device being used for intermittent chemotherapy may be flushed as infrequently as once monthly. Consult your institution's policy.

You should also read the heparin label carefully to make sure you're using the correct concentration of heparin for the flush. Heparin is manufactured in concentrations ranging from 10 units/ml to 20,000 units/ml (see *Heparin flushes*, page 150). A dilute concentration of heparin, ranging from 10 to 100 units/ml, may be used for flushes; the amount depends on the institution's policy and the type of venous access device being used. Concentrations stronger than 100 units/ml are contraindicated for this purpose because they can prolong a patient's clotting time. Some institutions have prefilled syringes of the correct concentration.

HEPARIN FLUSHES

Before using heparin to flush a venous access device, know your institution's policy on the correct heparin concentration to use—and read the label carefully. A dilute concentration of 10 to 100 units/ml may be used, but concentrations stronger than 100 units/ml are contraindicated for flushes.

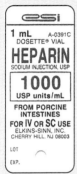

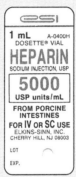

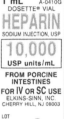

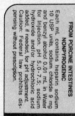

PRACTICE PROBLEMS

Prepared liquids

Check your answers against those on page 166.

1. A patient is to receive 1 mg of naloxone (Narcan) from a vial with this label:

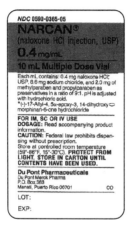

You would administer _____ ml.

2. A patient is to receive 10 mg of nalbuphine (Nubain) from a vial with this label:

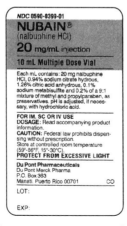

You would administer _____ ml.

3. A patient is to receive 5 mg of haloperidol (Haldol) from a vial with this label:

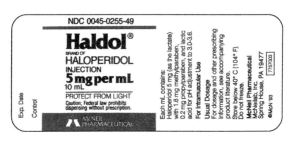

You would administer _____ ml.

4. A physician orders furosemide (Lasix) 40 mg I.V. push. An ampule of Lasix is labeled *10 mg/ml.* You would administer _____ ml.

5. A patient's Hickman catheter is to be flushed with 3 ml of heparin solution labeled *100 U/ml.* You would administer _____ units.

6. A physician orders 75 mg of meperidine (Demerol) I.M. A prefilled syringe containing 100 mg/2 ml is available. You would administer _____ ml.

7. A child is to receive 2.5 mg of diazepam (Valium) I.M. The vial is labeled *5 mg/5 ml.* You would administer _____ ml.

8. A physician orders atropine gr ¹⁄₁₅₀ I.M. The vial is labeled *0.4 mg/ml.* You would administer _____ ml.

9. A patient is to receive 5,000 units of heparin S.C. The vial is labeled *10,000 U/ml.* You would administer _____ ml.

10. A physician orders pentobarbital (Nembutal) 100 mg I.M. The ampule is labeled *50 mg/ml.* You would administer _____ ml.

Insulin

Check your answers against those on page 166.

1. A physician's order states *30 U NPH S.C.* Based on this information, you would draw up 30 units of

_____ in a _____ syringe.

2. A physician's order states *60 U regular beef insulin S.C.* Based on this information, you would draw up

_____ insulin in a _____ syringe.

3. A physician's order states *15 U regular human insulin plus 40 U NPH human insulin S.C.* Based on this information, you would use U-100 insulins and a _____ syringe and draw up the _____ insulin first.

4. Based on the following sliding scale order, you would administer _____ units of _____ insulin to a patient whose most recent blood glucose value is 300 mg/dl.

Blood glucose values	Insulin dose
< 180 mg/dl	No insulin
180 to 250 mg/dl	10 units regular insulin S.C.
251 to 390 mg/dl	20 units regular insulin S.C.
> 390 mg/dl	Call physician

5. Based on the chart above, you would draw up the U-100 insulin in a _____ syringe.

6. A physician's order states *Add 100 U of regular insulin to 500 ml of 0.45% saline solution, and infuse at 10 U/hr.* To do this, you would use a _____ syringe to draw up _____ units of regular insulin. You should set the infusion pump to deliver _____ ml/hr.

Reconstitution of a powder

Check your answers against those on page 166.

1. A patient is to receive 3.1 G ticarcillin (Timentin) I.V.P.B. The vial is labeled *Add 18.5 ml of diluent for 0.155 G/ml solution.* You would administer _____ ml.

2. A patient is to receive 1 G chloramphenicol (Chloromycetin) I.V.P.B. from a vial with this label:

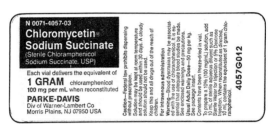

If reconstituted as directed, the concentration will be

_____ mg/ml, and the patient should receive

_____ ml.

3. A physician orders 1 G ampicillin (Polycillin-N) I.V.P.B. The vial is labeled:

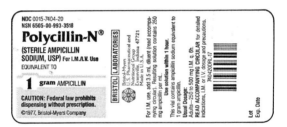

If 3.5 ml of diluent are added to the vial, you would withdraw

_____ ml of the prepared solution for the patient's dose.

4. The patient is to receive 500,000 units of penicillin G (Pfizerpen) from a vial with this label:

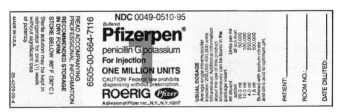

If 10 ml of diluent are added to the vial, the concentration

will be _____ units/ml, and the patient should receive _____ ml.

5. A physician orders 200,000 units penicillin G I.M. If a vial
with the same label as in the preceding question is used
and 20 ml of diluent is added, the concentration will be
_____units/ml, and the patient should receive
_____ ml.

6. A patient is to receive 500 mg cefazolin (Kefzol) I.V.P.B.
The vial is labeled *1 Gram Kefzol, add 3 ml diluent for solution
of 250 mg/ml.* You would administer _____ ml.

7. A physician orders methicillin (Staphcillin) 2 G I.V.P.B.,
and 1-G vials are available. A 1-G vial requires 5 ml of diluent
to produce a 200 mg/ml solution. You would administer
_____ ml.

8. A child is to receive 400 mg of ceftazidime (Fortaz)
I.V.P.B. The vial is labeled *1 G Fortaz, add 10 ml diluent for
100 mg/ml solution.* You would administer _____ ml.

9. A child is to receive 1 G mezlocillin (Mezlin) I.V.P.B. A 2-
G vial is labeled *Add 20 ml diluent for 100 mg/ml solution.* You
would administer _____ ml.

10. A physician orders ticarcillin (Ticar) 2 G I.V.P.B. q6h. The
vials are labeled *1 Gram Ticar. Add 2 ml diluent for
500 mg/ml solution.* You would administer _____ ml.

Large-volume infusions
Check your answers against those on page 167.

1. The physician orders 2,000 ml of D₅LR I.V. over the first
24 hours postoperatively. You have an administration
set with a drip factor of 15 gtt/ml, so you set it
to deliver _____ gtt/minute.

2. A patient is to receive 1 L of I.V. lactated Ringer's solution over 10 hours. A set with a drip factor of 10 gtt/ml is to be used. The rate should be set at _____ gtt/minute.

3. A patient is to receive 1,000 ml of D_5NSS over 4 hours. Using a set with a drip factor of 20 gtt/ml, the flow rate should be _____ gtt/minute.

4. If a patient's I.V. infusion is dripping at 31 gtt/minute and the set has a drip factor of 15 gtt/ml, the patient will receive _____ ml during your 8-hour shift.

5. The physician orders I.V. $D_5\frac{1}{3}NS$ at 80 ml/hour. A set with a drip factor of 20 gtt/ml is to be used. The rate should be set at _____ gtt/minute.

6. If a child is to receive 30 ml/hr of $D_50.25NS$ I.V. and you are using a minidrip delivery set, you will use a drip rate of _____ gtt/minute.

7. If a patient is to receive 500 ml of $D_50.45NS$ I.V. over 24 hours and a microdrip set is used, the drip rate will be _____ gtt/minute.

8. If a patient is to receive a maintenance I.V. at 15 gtt/minute using a micropdrip set over an 8-hour period, the intake will equal _____ ml.

9. The physician's order reads *Administer 1,000 ml $D_50.45NSS$ c̄ 40 mEq of KCl over 6 hrs.* You have a set with a drip factor of 15. The drip rate should be _____ gtt/minute.

10. If a patient is to receive 100 ml/hr I.V. and the drip factor is 15, you will need to set the drip rate at _____ gtt/minute.

Fluid replacement
Check your answers against those on page 167.
(*Note:* For problems 1-5, a shift is 8 hours)

1. The physician orders I.V. NS for a ml/ml replacement of chest tube drainage each shift, and I.V. D_5NS at 125 ml/hour.

The chest tube drained 400 ml to be replaced over this shift. The drip factor for both sets is 20 gtt/ml. The NS should be set at _____ gtt/minute, and the D₅NS should be set at _____ gtt/minute.

2. A patient is to have one half the nasogastric drainage on the previous shift replaced during this shift with I.V. NS, and I.V. D₅½NS at 80 ml/hour. If the nasogastric drainage was 700 ml and the drip factor for the NS is 20 gtt/ml and for the D₅½NS is 15 gtt/ml, the NS should infuse at _____ gtt/minute, and the D₅½NS should infuse at _____ gtt/minute.

3. The physician orders I.V. NS for a ml/ml replacement of intestinal tube drainage per shift, and I.V. lactated Ringer's solution at 100 ml/hour. The intestinal tube drained 200 ml to be replaced over this shift. The drip factor for the NS is 60 gtt/ml and for the lactated Ringer's is 15 gtt/ml. The NS should be set at _____ gtt/minute, and the lactated Ringer's at _____ gtt/minute.

4. A patient is to receive I.V. NS to replace the chest tube drainage of the previous shift, and 1 L D₅NS over 10 hours. If the chest tube drained 300 ml and the drip factor for the NS is 60 gtt/ml and for the D₅NS is 10 gtt/ml, the NS should infuse at _____ gtt/minute, and the D₅NS should infuse at _____ gtt/minute.

5. The physician orders I.V. NS with 20 mEq KCl/L to replace one-half the nasogastric tube drainage per shift, and I.V. lactated Ringer's solution at 75 ml/hour. The nasogastric tube drained 800 ml during the last shift. The drip factor for both the NS and the lactated Ringer's is 20 gtt/ml. The NS should be set at _____ gtt/minute and the lactated Ringer's at _____ gtt/minute.

Fluid challenges
Check your answers against those on page 167.

1. The physician orders a 200 ml I.V. fluid challenge over 30 minutes, followed by a regular infusion rate of 100 ml/hour. If the drip factor is 10 gtt/ml, the fluid bolus will run at _____ gtt/minute, and the regular I.V. will run at _____ gtt/minute.

2. A patient is to receive 400 ml I.V. NS over 1 hour, followed by I.V. NS at 50 ml/hour. The set has a drip factor of 15 gtt/ml. For the first hour, the I.V. rate would be _____ gtt/minute. After the first hour, the I.V. rate would be _____ gtt/minute.

3. The physician orders a 300 ml I.V. fluid challenge over 30 minutes, followed by a regular infusion rate of 1 L over 10 hours. If the drip factor is 10 gtt/ml, the fluid bolus will run at _____ gtt/minute, and the regular I.V. will run at _____ gtt/minute.

4. A patient is to receive 200 ml I.V. NS over 15 minutes, followed by I.V. NS at 100 ml/hour. The set has a drip factor of 10 gtt/ml. For the first 15 minutes, the I.V. rate would be _____ gtt/minute. After the first 15 minutes, the I.V. rate would be _____ gtt/minute.

5. The physician orders a 250 ml I.V. fluid challenge over 30 minutes, followed by a regular infusion rate of 75 ml/hour. If the drip factor is 10 gtt/ml, the fluid bolus will run at _____ gtt/minute, and the regular I.V. will run at_____ gtt/minute.

Medication additives
Check your answers against those on page 167.

1. A physician orders 20,000 units of heparin in 500 ml D$_5$W to infuse at 25 ml/hour. The dose will be _____ units/hour.

2. A patient is to receive 1,200 units/hour of heparin. Using a solution of 10,000 units of heparin in 250 ml D_5W, the infuser pump should be set at _____ ml/hour.

3. A physician orders 20,000 units heparin in 500 ml D_5W to infuse at 1,500 units/hour. The infuser pump should be set at _____ ml/hour.

4. A patient is to receive a solution of 20,000 units of heparin in 500 ml D_5W at a rate of 34 ml/hour. The patient will receive _____ units in 24 hours.

5. A physician orders 20,000 units of heparin in 250 ml D_5W to infuse at 16 ml/hour. The patient will receive _____ units/hour.

6. A child is to receive 250 mg aminophylline in 250 ml D_5W at a rate of 20 ml/hour. The patient will receive _____ mg/hour.

7. A physician orders 500 mg aminophylline in 250 ml D_5W to infuse at 34 mg/hour. The infuser pump should be set at _____ ml/hour.

8. A patient is to receive 500 mg aminophylline in 500 ml D_5W at a rate of 28 ml/hour. The patient will receive _____ mg/hour.

9. A physician orders 500 mg aminophylline in 250 ml D_5W to infuse at a rate of 20 ml/hour. The patient will receive _____ mg/hour.

10. A patient is to receive 250 mg aminophylline in 250 ml D_5W at 32 mg/hour. The infuser pump should be set at _____ ml/hour.

Medication additives: Critical care
Check your answers against those on page 168.

1. If a solution contains 400 mg dopamine in 250 ml D_5W, each milliliter of the solution will contain _____ mg and _____ mcg of dopamine.

2. If a patient weighing 65 kg is to receive 5 mcg/kg/minute of the above dopamine infusion, the patient should receive _____ mcg/minute and _____ ml/minute. The infusion pump should be set at _____ ml/hour.

3. A physician has ordered 50 mg of nitroprusside mixed in 250 ml of D_5W. The patient weighs 70 kg and is to receive an infusion of 3 mcg/kg/minute. The solution concentration is _____ mcg/ml. The patient should receive _____ mcg/minute. The infusion rate should be _____ ml/hour.

4. A patient is to receive 2 mg/minute of bretylium. The solution contains 500 mg of bretylium in 50 ml of D_5W. The solution concentration is _____ mg/ml. The patient should receive _____ mg/hour, and the flow rate should be _____ ml/hour.

5. A physician has ordered 250 ml of D_5W with 500 mg of dobutamine hydrochloride. The patient weighs 150 lb and is to receive an infusion of 6 mcg/kg/minute. The patient weighs _____ kg and should receive _____ mg/minute. The infusion pump should be set at _____ ml/hour.

6. A physician orders a lidocaine drip at 4 mg/minute. The I.V. solution is 500 ml of D_5W with 2 G of lidocaine. To infuse the drug at 4 mg/minute, the flow rate should be _____ ml/minute, or _____ ml/hour.

7. A patient weighing 176 lb is receiving a dopamine infusion at 0.5 ml/minute. The solution contains 250 mg of dopamine in 500 ml D_5W. The concentration of the

solution is _____ mg/ml, and the patient will
receive _____ mg/minute. The patient weighs
_____ kg and will receive _____
mcg/kg/minute.

8. A patient weighing 165 lb is receiving an infusion of 50
mg of nitroprusside mixed in 250 ml of D_5W. The I.V. solution
is infusing at 0.5 ml/minute to keep the patient's systolic
blood pressure at less than 160 mm Hg. The patient weighs
_____ kg. The concentration of nitroprusside in
the solution is _____ mcg/ml. The patient will be
receiving _____ mcg/kg/minute.

9. If a patient is receiving lidocaine in a 2:1 concentration at
60 ml/hour, the solution concentration is _____
mg/ml of lidocaine, and the dose received will be
_____ mg/hour.

10. The safe maximum dosage for dobutamine is 10 mcg/kg/min-
ute. A patient weighing 85 kg is receiving a 4:1 solution of it.
The solution's concentration is _____ mg/ml.
The patient could safely receive up to _____ mg/min-
ute, which would be a rate of _____ ml/hour.

Medication additives: Obstetrics
Check your answers against those on page 168.

1. A solution contains 10 units of oxytocin in 500 ml NS. The
concentration of the solution is _____ units/ml, or
_____ milliunits/ml.

2. A patient is to receive 0.75 G/hour of magnesium sulfate.
The 500-ml bottle of D_5W contains 8 G of the drug. The concentration of the solution is _____ mg/ml. It
should be infused at _____ ml/hour.

3. The physician's order states *10 U Pitocin in 1,000 ml NS; infuse at 4 mU/minute*. The concentration of the solution is _____ milliunits/ml. It should be infused at _____ ml/minute, or _____ ml/hour.

4. The physician orders 500 mg/hour of $MgSO_4$. The 500-ml I.V. bottle contains 4 G of the drug. The concentration of the solution is _____ mg/ml. The infusion rate is _____ ml/hour.

5. A patient is to receive oxytocin as follows: 4 milliunits/minute for 20 minutes, followed by 6 milliunits/minute for 20 minutes. The label on the 500-ml bag of NSS reads *oxytocin 10 units*. The concentration of the solution is _____ milliunits/ml. The infusion pump should be set at _____ ml/hour for the first 20 minutes and _____ ml/hour for the next 20 minutes.

Small-volume infusions

Check your answers against those on page 168.

1. A patient is to receive 50 ml of an I.V. vancomycin solution over 30 minutes. The set has a drip factor of 10 gtt/ml. The drip rate will be _____ gtt/minute.

2. The physician orders phenytoin 300 mg I.V.P.B. q8h. The medication is diluted in 100 ml NS to infuse over 30 minutes. If the drip factor is 15 gtt/ml, the rate should be set at _____ gtt/minute.

3. A patient is to receive 100 ml of an I.V. penicillin solution over 45 minutes. The set has a drip factor of 10 gtt/ml. The drip rate will be _____ gtt/minute.

4. The physician orders 1 G cefazolin I.V.P.B. q8h. The medication is diluted in 50 ml D_5W to infuse over 15 minutes. If the drip factor is 20 gtt/ml, the rate should be set at _____ gtt/minute.

5. A patient is to receive 50 ml of an I.V. gentamicin solution over 1 hour. The set has a microdrip. The drip rate will be _____ gtt/minute.

6. The physician orders methyldopa 250 mg I.V.P.B. q6h. The medication is diluted in 100 ml D_5W to infuse over 1 hour. If the drip factor is 15 gtt/ml, the rate should be set at _____ gtt/minute.

7. A patient is to receive 10 ml of an I.V. dexamethasone solution over 10 minutes. The set has a drip factor of 20 gtt/ml. The drip rate will be _____ gtt/minute.

8. The physician orders 2 G ceftriaxone I.V.P.B. q.d. The medication is diluted in 150 ml D_5W to infuse over 60 minutes. If the drip factor is 15 gtt/ml, the rate should be set at _____ gtt/minute.

9. A patient is to receive 100 ml of an I.V. cefoperazone solution over 1 hour. The set has a drip factor of 20 gtt/ml. The drip rate will be _____ gtt/minute.

10. The physician orders doxycycline 200 mg I.V.P.B. q.d. The medication is diluted in 150 ml D_5W to infuse over 1½ hours. The set has a drip factor of 15 gtt/ml. The rate should be set at _____ gtt/minute.

Blood transfusions

Check your answers against those on pages 168 and 169.

1. The patient is to receive 275 ml of packed RBCs over 2 hours. The set has a drip factor of 10 gtt/ml. The drip rate of the transfusion should be _____ gtt/minute.

2. The physician orders 1 unit of packed RBCs to infuse over 4 hours. The unit contains 250 ml, and the set has a drip factor of 15 gtt/ml. The drip rate should be _____ gtt/minute.

3. The patient is to receive 100 ml of platelets over 15 minutes. The set has a drip factor of 15 gtt/ml. The drip rate of the transfusion should be _____ gtt/minute.

4. The physician orders 1 unit of whole blood to infuse over 3 hours. The unit contains 250 ml, and the set has a drip factor of 15 gtt/ml. The drip rate should be _____ gtt/minute.

5. The patient is to receive 50 ml of platelets over 10 minutes. The set has a drip factor of 10 gtt/ml. The drip rate of the transfusion should be _____ gtt/minute.

6. The physician orders 1 unit of packed RBCs to infuse over 2½ hours. The unit contains 275 ml, and the set has a drip factor of 15 gtt/ml. The drip rate should be _____ gtt/minute.

7. The patient is to receive 100 ml of cryoprecipitate over 30 minutes. The set has a drip factor of 10 gtt/ml. The drip rate of the cryoprecipitate should be _____ gtt/minute.

8. The physician orders 1 unit of whole blood to infuse over 3 hours. The unit contains 275 ml, and the set has a drip factor of 10 gtt/ml. The drip rate should be _____ gtt/minute.

9. The patient is to receive 125 ml of cryoprecipitate over 45 minutes. The set has a drip factor of 15 gtt/ml. The drip rate of the transfusion should be _____ gtt/minute.

10. The physician orders 1 unit of packed RBCs to infuse over 2 hours. The unit contains 250 ml, and the set has a drip factor of 10 gtt/ml. The drip rate should be _____ gtt/minute.

Patient-controlled analgesia
Check your answers against those on page 169.

1. After 4 hours, the nurse checks a patient's PCA log and notes that the patient requested and received three doses of

1 ml each. The nurse notes that each milliliter contains 1 mg of morphine. The patient received _____ mg of morphine in 4 hours.

2. At the beginning of the shift, the nurse notes that 30 ml of medication remain in a patient's PCA device. The record shows that 2 mg of morphine per milliliter was placed in the device. After 2 hours, the nurse checks the PCA log and notes that the patient made six attempts and received five doses of 1 ml each. The nurse calculates that the patient received _____ mg of morphine in 2 hours.

3. After 4 hours, the nurse checks a patient's PCA log and notes that he requested and received 3 doses of 1 ml each. The nurse notes that each milliliter contains 0.5 mg of morphine. The patient received _____ mg of morphine in 4 hours.

4. At the beginning of the shift, the nurse notes that 30 ml of medication remain in a patient's PCA device. The machine is set to deliver 1 ml per dose. The nurse checks the PCA log after 4 hours, noting that the patient has made eight attempts and received seven doses of medication. At the end of the next 4 hours, the patient has made six attempts and received six doses of medication. At the end of the 8-hour shift, how many milliliters of medication remain in the PCA device?

5. At the beginning of the shift, the nurse notes that 22 ml of medication remain in a patient's PCA device. The machine is set to deliver 2 ml per dose. The nurse notes that 1 ml of fluid contains 1 mg of morphine. After 4 hours, the patient has made five attempts and received five doses. The nurse notes on the medication record that the patient received _____ mg of morphine and that _____ ml of fluid remain in the PCA device.

ANSWERS TO PRACTICE PROBLEMS

Prepared liquids

1. 2.5 ml
2. 0.5 ml
3. 1 ml
4. 4 ml
5. 300 units
6. 1.5 ml
7. 2.5 ml
8. 1 ml
9. 0.5 ml
10. 2 ml

Insulin

1. NPH insulin 100 units/ml (U-100) in a U-100 syringe
2. 60 units of regular beef U-100 insulin in a U-100 syringe
3. U-100 syringe; regular insulin first
4. 20 units of regular insulin S.C.
5. U-100 syringe
6. U-100 syringe; 100 units; 50 ml/hour

Reconstitution of a powder

1. 20 ml
2. 100 mg/ml; 10 ml
3. 4 ml
4. 100,000 units/ml; 5 ml
5. 50,000 units/ml; 4 ml
6. 2 ml
7. 10 ml (use two 1-G vials; use 5 ml from each vial)
8. 4 ml
9. 10 ml
10. 4 ml (use two 1-G vials; use 2 ml from each vial)

Large-volume infusions

1. 21 gtt/minute
2. 17 gtt/minute
3. 83 gtt/minute
4. 1,000 ml
5. 27 gtt/minute
6. 30 gtt/minute
7. 21 gtt/minute
8. 120 ml
9. 42 gtt/minute
10. 25 gtt/minute

Fluid replacement

1. 17 gtt/minute; 42 gtt/minute
2. 15 gtt/minute; 20 gtt/minute
3. 25 gtt/minute; 25 gtt/minute
4. 38 gtt/minute; 17 gtt/minute
5. 17 gtt/minute; 25 gtt/minute

Fluid challenges

1. 67 gtt/minute; 17 gtt/minute
2. 100 gtt/minute; 13 gtt/minute
3. 100 gtt/minute; 17 gtt/minute
4. 133 gtt/minute; 17 gtt/minute
5. 83 gtt/minute; 13 gtt/minute

Medication additives

1. 1,000 units/hour
2. 30 ml/hour
3. 38 ml/hour
4. 32,640 units
5. 1,280 units/hour
6. 20 mg/hour
7. 17 ml/hour
8. 28 mg/hour
9. 40 mg/hour
10. 32 ml/hour

Medication additives: Critical care

1. 1.6 mg/ml; 1,600 mcg/ml
2. 325 mcg/minute; 0.2 ml/minute; 12 ml/hour
3. 200 mcg/ml; 210 mcg/minute; 63 ml/hour
4. 10 mg/ml; 120 mg/hour; 12 ml/hour
5. 68.2 kg; 0.4 mg/minute; 12 ml/hour
6. 1 ml/minute; 60 ml/hour
7. 0.5 mg/ml; 0.25 mg/minute; 80 kg; 3.1 mcg/kg/minute
8. 75 kg; 200 mcg/ml; 1.33 mcg/kg/minute
9. 2 mg/ml; 120 mg/hour
10. 4 mg/ml; 0.85 mg/minute; 13 ml/hour

Medication additives: Obstetrics

1. 0.02 units/ml; 20 milliunits/ml
2. 16 mg/ml; 47 ml/hour
3. 10 milliunits/ml; 0.4 ml/minute; 24 ml/hour
4. 8 mg/ml; 63 ml/hour
5. 20 milliunits/ml; 12 ml/hour; 18 ml/hour

Small-volume infusions

1. 17 gtt/minute
2. 50 gtt/minute
3. 22 gtt/minute
4. 67 gtt/minute
5. 50 gtt/minute
6. 25 gtt/minute
7. 20 gtt/minute
8. 38 gtt/minute
9. 33 gtt/minute
10. 25 gtt/minute

Blood transfusions

1. 23 gtt/minute
2. 16 gtt/minute
3. 100 gtt/minute
4. 21 gtt/minute

5. 50 gtt/minute
6. 28 gtt/minute
7. 33 gtt/minute
8. 15 gtt/minute
9. 42 gtt/minute
10. 21 gtt/minute

Patient-controlled analgesia

1. 3 mg
2. 10 mg
3. 5.5 mg
4. 17 ml
5. 10 mg; 12 ml

SOLUTIONS, OINTMENTS, AND PATCHES

This chapter provides information about calculations for concentrations of enteral and topical solutions and for topical ointments and patches.

PREPARATION OF SOLUTIONS

A *solution* is a liquid preparation that contains a *solute* (a liquid or solid form of a drug or nutritional supplement) dissolved in a *solvent* (diluent), usually water, sterile water, normal saline solution, or dextrose 5% in water. Solutions used internally include enteral feeding solutions administered orally or via nasogastric, gastrostomy, or jejunostomy tubes and parenteral solutions such as intravenous fluids. Solutions used externally include topical solutions to irrigate wounds or to apply to the body as soaks. Solutions intended for external use should never be administered internally.

Solutions come in different strengths, or concentrations, which can be expressed as *percentage* or *ratio* solutions. The concentration of a solution is calculated in the same way whether the solution is intended for internal or external use. This chapter describes percentage and ratio solutions and applies this information in patient situations for enteral solutions and topical solutions. Patient situations for parenteral solutions are discussed in Chapter 5, Calculating Parenteral Drug Dosages.

Percentage solutions

The clearest and most common way to label or describe a solution is as a percentage. This is also the easiest to use when making dosage calculations, dilutions, or alterations. A percentage solution may be expressed in terms of weight/volume (W/V) or volume/volume (V/V). In a W/V percentage solution, the percentage, or strength, refers to the number of grams of solute (weight) per 100 ml of finished solution (volume). In a V/V percentage solution, the percentage, or strength, refers to the number of milliliters of solute (volume) per 100 ml of finished solution (volume). This relationship can be expressed mathematically as:

%(W/V) = grams solute/100 ml finished solution

%(V/V) = milliliters solute/100 ml finished solution

This mathematical relationship lets you know the contents of any percentage solution by reading its label, as shown in *Contents of percentage solutions,* page 172.

Ratio solutions
The strength of a ratio solution is usually expressed as two numbers separated by a colon. The first number in the ratio signifies the amount of a drug in grams (in a W/V solution) or in milliliters (in a V/V solution). The second number indicates the volume of finished solution in milliliters. This relationship can be expressed as:

ratio = amount of drug : amount of finished solution

See *Contents of ratio solutions,* page 173, for more information.

Any ratio solution can be converted to a percentage solution, using the ratio and proportion method. For example, if you wanted to convert the Burow's solution in the chart to a percentage solution, you would use the ratio 1 G:40 ml in a proportion with the unknown quantity and a finished solution of 100 ml:

$$1 \text{ G}:40 \text{ ml} :: \text{X G}:100 \text{ ml}$$

$$40 \text{ ml} \times \text{X G} = 1 \text{ G} \times 100 \text{ ml}$$

$$\text{X} = \frac{1 \text{ G} \times 100 \text{ ml}}{40 \text{ ml}}$$

$$\text{X} = 2.5 \text{ G}$$

$$\text{X} = 2.5\%$$

Dosage calculations with solutions

You may need to prepare solutions or alter them by adding more solute to increase their concentration or by adding more solvent (diluent) to decrease their concentration. If you know a solution's

CONTENTS OF PERCENTAGE SOLUTIONS

You can determine the contents of a W/V or V/V percentage solution by reading the label, as shown below.

PERCENTAGE SOLUTION	CONTENTS
5% (W/V) boric acid solution	5 G of boric acid in 100 ml of finished solution
0.9% (W/V) NaCl	0.9 G of sodium chloride in 100 ml of finished solution
5% (W/V) dextrose	5 G of dextrose in 100 ml of finished solution
2% (V/V) hydrogen peroxide	2 ml of hydrogen peroxide in 100 ml of finished solution
70% (V/V) isopropyl alcohol	70 ml of isopropyl alcohol in 100 ml of finished solution
10% (V/V) glycerin	10 ml of glycerin in 100 ml of finished solution

concentration, you can use the following guidelines to calculate any necessary changes:

■ Convert the known units of measure to the same system (all metric, household, or apothecaries'), if necessary.

■ Determine the concentration on hand and the unknowns in the desired concentration. When using a pure powder or solid as a solute, assume the concentration is 100% unless otherwise stated. Also assume that a saturated solution or pure liquid concentrate has a concentration of 100% unless otherwise stated.

■ Set up the necessary ratios or fractions and solve for unknown quantities. When preparing a percentage solution by adding solutes to solvents, use one of these proportions:

Ratio approach

weaker : stronger :: solute : solvent

or

small % strength : large % strength :: small volume : large volume

CONTENTS OF RATIO SOLUTIONS

You can determine the contents of a W/V or V/V ratio solution from the label, as shown below.

RATIO SOLUTION	CONTENTS
benzalkonium chloride 1:750	1 G of benzalkonium chloride in 750 ml of finished solution
silver nitrate 1:100	1 G of silver nitrate in 100 ml of finished solution
epinephrine (Adrenalin) 1:1,000	1 G of epinephrine in 1,000 ml of finished solution
Burow's solution (aluminum acetate) 1:40	1 G of aluminum acetate in 40 ml of finished solution

Fraction approach

$$\frac{\text{weaker}}{\text{stronger}} = \frac{\text{solute}}{\text{solvent}}$$

or

$$\frac{\text{small \% strength}}{\text{large \% strength}} = \frac{\text{small volume}}{\text{large volume}}$$

■ Adjust the amount of diluent to obtain the correct total volume. Although a solid combined with a diluent often increases the total volume of the prepared solution, the increase is usually insignificant and need not be considered in calculations. The increase, however, will be significant and should be considered when adding either a large amount of solid or a small amount of diluent. When adding a liquid, subtract its volume from the total volume desired. The calculation tells the volume of diluent to add. For example, if the preparation of 1 L of solution requires 50 ml of a liquid drug, add the 50 ml of liquid drug to 950 ml of diluent.

Patient situations: Enteral solutions

1. A physician orders 8 oz of a 0.9% (W/V) saline solution (sodium chloride in water) as a gargle. How many grams of sodium chloride should you include in the solution?

■ First, convert all units of measure to the same system, using the conversion factor 1 oz = 30 ml to change 8 oz to milliliters:

$$8 \text{ oz}:X \text{ ml} :: 1 \text{ oz}:30 \text{ ml}$$

$$X \text{ ml} \times 1 \text{ oz} = 8 \text{ oz} \times 30 \text{ ml}$$

$$X = \frac{8 \text{ oz} \times 30 \text{ ml}}{1 \text{ oz}}$$

$$X = 240 \text{ ml solution required}$$

■ Next, determine the strength of the desired solution, based on its percentage:

$$0.9\% \text{ (W/V) sodium chloride} = 0.9 \text{ G}/100 \text{ ml}$$

■ Set up the proportion to determine the amount of sodium chloride needed to prepare 240 ml of the desired solution:

$$0.9 \text{ G}:100 \text{ ml} :: X \text{ G}:240 \text{ ml}$$

$$100 \text{ ml} \times X \text{ G} = 0.9 \text{ G} \times 240 \text{ ml}$$

$$X = \frac{0.9 \text{ G} \times 240 \text{ ml}}{100 \text{ ml}}$$

$$X = 2.16 \text{ or } 2.2 \text{ G sodium chloride}$$

Thus, you'll need 2.2 G of sodium chloride to prepare the ordered solution.

2. You must prepare 500 ml of a 1:2 nutritional replacement solution for a nasogastric feeding. How much nutritional replacement and water do you need?

■ Set up a proportion with the known and unknown quantities (V/V):

$$\frac{1 \text{ volume nutritional replacement}}{2 \text{ volumes finished solution}} = \frac{X \text{ ml}}{500 \text{ ml}}$$

■ Solve for X to determine the amount of nutritional replacement to use:

$$X \text{ ml} \times 2 \text{ volumes} = 500 \text{ ml} \times 1 \text{ volume}$$

$$X = \frac{500 \text{ ml} \times 1}{2}$$

$$X = 250 \text{ ml}$$

■ Subtract to determine the amount of water to add:

$$
\begin{array}{rl}
500 \text{ ml} & \text{finished solution} \\
- \ 250 \text{ ml} & \text{nutritional replacement} \\
\hline
250 \text{ ml} & \text{water}
\end{array}
$$

Thus, to prepare 500 ml of a 1:2 nutritional replacement solution, you should mix 250 ml of nutritional replacement with 250 ml of water.

3. A drug order requires you to administer 15 G of acetylcysteine as a 5% oral solution. You must prepare the 5% solution from a 20% stock solution on hand. How many milliliters of the stock solution do you need? How many milliliters of diluent should you use?

▪ Determine the stock solution's strength based on its percentage:

$$20\% \text{ (W/V) acetylcysteine} = 20 \text{ G}/100 \text{ ml}$$

▪ Set up a proportion to calculate how much stock solution will yield 15 G:

$$20 \text{ G}{:}100 \text{ ml} :: 15 \text{ G}{:}X \text{ ml}$$

$$100 \text{ ml} \times 15 \text{ G} = 20 \text{ G} \times X \text{ ml}$$

$$X = \frac{100 \text{ ml} \times 15 \text{ G}}{20 \text{ G}}$$

$$X = 75 \text{ ml}$$

▪ Determine the desired solution's strength based on its percentage:

$$5\% \text{ (W/V) acetylcysteine} = 5 \text{ G}/100 \text{ ml}$$

▪ Set up a proportion to calculate the total volume of finished solution if the concentration is 5%:

$$15 \text{ G}{:}X \text{ ml} :: 5 \text{ G}{:}100 \text{ ml}$$

$$X \text{ ml} \times 5 \text{ G} = 15 \text{ G} \times 100 \text{ ml}$$

$$X = \frac{15 \text{ G} \times 100 \text{ ml}}{5 \text{ G}}$$

$$X = 300 \text{ ml}$$

▪ Subtract to determine the amount of diluent to add:

$$\begin{array}{rl} 300 \text{ ml} & \text{finished 5\% solution (total volume)} \\ - 75 \text{ ml} & \text{20\% solution needed} \\ \hline 225 \text{ ml} & \text{diluent to add} \end{array}$$

Thus, you should mix 75 ml of the 20% stock solution with 225 ml of diluent to prepare the 5% solution ordered.

Patient situations: Topical solutions

1. You need to prepare 200 ml of a 10% magnesium sulfate (Epsom salts) solution to use as a soak. Because magnesium sulfate comes in a pure powder, you can assume that its strength is 100%. How many grams of magnesium sulfate do you need?

■ Because the units of measure already appear in the same system, begin by determining the strength of the desired solution, based on its percentage:

$$10\% \text{ (W/V) magnesium sulfate} = 10 \text{ G}/100 \text{ ml}$$

■ Set up a proportion with the desired quantity (200 ml) and strength:

$$10 \text{ G}:100 \text{ ml} :: X \text{ G}:200 \text{ ml}$$

$$100 \text{ ml} \times X = 10 \text{ G} \times 200 \text{ ml}$$

$$X = \frac{10 \text{ G} \times 200 \text{ ml}}{100 \text{ ml}}$$

$$X = 20 \text{ G}$$

Thus, you'll need 20 G of magnesium sulfate to prepare the solution.

2. You must prepare 50 ml of a 10% (V/V) solution of glycerin in water. How much pure glycerin liquid and water should you use?

■ Determine the solution's strength based on its percentage:

$$10\% \text{ (V/V) glycerin} = 10 \text{ ml}/100 \text{ ml}$$

■ Set up a proportion with the known and unknown quantities:

$$10 \text{ ml}:100 \text{ ml} :: X \text{ ml}:50 \text{ ml}$$

$$100 \text{ ml} \times X \text{ ml} = 10 \text{ ml} \times 50 \text{ ml}$$

$$X = \frac{10 \text{ ml} \times 50 \text{ ml}}{100 \text{ ml}}$$

$$X = 5 \text{ ml of glycerin}$$

■ Subtract to determine the amount of water to add:

$$
\begin{array}{rl}
50 \text{ ml} & \text{finished solution (total volume)} \\
-5 \text{ ml} & \text{glycerin volume} \\
\hline
45 \text{ ml} & \text{water to add}
\end{array}
$$

Thus, to prepare 50 ml of a 10% glycerin in water solution, you need 5 ml of glycerin and 45 ml of water.

3. You must prepare 1,000 ml of a 1% (W/V) sterile kanamycin irrigation solution from 250 mg/ml of on-hand kanamycin injection. How much kanamycin and sterile water should you use?

■ Determine the desired solution's strength based on its percentage:

$$1\% \text{ (W/V) kanamycin} = 1 \text{ G}/100 \text{ ml}$$

■ Set up a proportion with this information to determine the amount of kanamycin needed:

$$1 \text{ G}:100 \text{ ml} :: \text{X G}:1{,}000 \text{ ml}$$

$$100 \text{ ml} \times \text{X G} = 1 \text{ G} \times 1{,}000 \text{ ml}$$

$$\text{X} = \frac{1 \text{ G} \times 1{,}000 \text{ ml}}{100 \text{ ml}}$$

$$\text{X} = 10 \text{ G}$$

■ Convert this to milligrams to use the same units of measure:

$$10 \text{ G} = 10{,}000 \text{ mg}$$

■ Set up a proportion to calculate the volume of kanamycin injection needed to deliver 10,000 mg:

$$250 \text{ mg}:1 \text{ ml} :: 10{,}000 \text{ mg}:\text{X ml}$$

$$1 \text{ ml} \times 10{,}000 \text{ mg} = 250 \text{ mg} \times \text{X ml}$$

$$\text{X} = \frac{1 \text{ ml} \times 10{,}000 \text{ mg}}{250 \text{ mg}}$$

$$\text{X} = 40 \text{ ml}$$

■ Subtract to determine the amount of sterile water to add:

$$\begin{array}{rl} 1{,}000 \text{ ml} & \text{finished solution (total volume)} \\ - \quad 40 \text{ ml} & \text{kanamycin injection needed} \\ \hline 960 \text{ ml} & \text{water to add} \end{array}$$

Thus, to prepare 1,000 ml of a 1% kanamycin irrigation solution, you need to mix 40 ml of kanamycin with 960 ml of sterile water.

4. From a 3% stock solution, you must prepare 100 ml of a 2% hexachlorophene solution. How much hexachlorophene and water do you need?

■ Determine the strength of the stock and desired solutions based on their percentages:

$$3\% \text{ (W/V) stock solution} = 3 \text{ G}/100 \text{ ml}$$

$$2\% \text{ (W/V) desired solution} = 2 \text{ G}/100 \text{ ml}$$

■ Set up a proportion with this information to determine the amount of stock solution needed:

$$2 \text{ G}:\text{X ml} :: 3 \text{ G}:100 \text{ ml}$$

$$\text{X ml} \times 3 \text{ G} = 2 \text{ G} \times 100 \text{ ml}$$

$$\text{X} = \frac{2 \text{ G} \times 100 \text{ ml}}{3 \text{ G}}$$

$$\text{X} = 66.7 \text{ or } 67 \text{ ml}$$

■ Subtract to determine the amount of water to add:

$$
\begin{array}{rl}
100\ ml & \text{finished solution (total volume)} \\
-\quad 67\ ml & \text{3\% stock solution needed} \\
\hline
33\ ml & \text{water to add}
\end{array}
$$

Thus, to prepare 100 ml of a 2% hexachlorophene solution, you would mix 67 ml of a 3% hexachlorophene solution with 33 ml of water.

TOPICAL OINTMENTS AND PATCHES

When a physician orders ointments as part of wound care or as dermatologic treatment, the amount to apply is usually left to the nurse's judgment, occasionally with such general guidance as "use a thin layer" or "thickly apply." When an ointment contains a medication intended for a visceral effect, more specific administration guidelines are necessary. Several medications that act on the cardiovascular system are applied topically.

USING A PAPER RULER APPLICATOR

To measure a specified amount of ointment from a tube, squeeze the ordered length of ointment (in inches or centimeters) onto a paper ruler like the one shown here. Then use the ruler to apply the ointment to the patient's skin at the ordered time, following the pharmaceutical manufacturer's guidelines for administration.

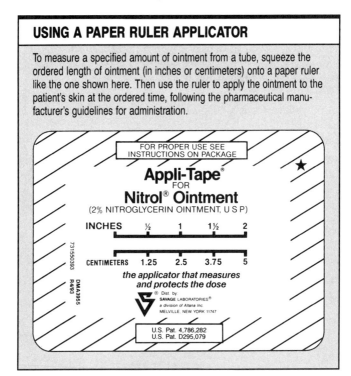

Nitroglycerin ointment, used to treat angina, is available in sustained-release transdermal patches that contain the ointment and in tubes from which you measure the correct dose. To apply a transdermal patch of nitroglycerin, remove the previously applied patch and replace it with the new patch at the ordered time, following the pharmaceutical manufacturer's guidelines for administration. To apply ointment from a tube, you'll use a paper ruler applicator, as shown in *Using a paper ruler applicator.*

The fentanyl transdermal system (Duragesic patch) also is applied topically, but is used to manage chronic pain. The fentanyl patch holds the drug in a reservoir behind a membrane that allows controlled drug absorption through the skin. It is available in 25, 50, 75, and 100 mcg/hour; the higher dosages are used for opioid-resistant patients. To ensure that the patient receives the correct dosage, change the patch every 72 hours, check the label to verify the fentanyl dosage, and note the size and color of the patch. Patch size increases and patch color changes as the dosage increases.

PRACTICE PROBLEMS

Enteral solutions
The answers to these problems follow on page 181.

1. A patient is to have a 25% solution of Ensure for a nasogastric feeding. A 250-ml can of Ensure is available. You should mix the can of Ensure with _____ ml of water.

2. The physician orders 500 ml of a 1:2 Isocal solution for a gastrostomy feeding. You should use _____ ml of Isocal and _____ ml of water.

3. A patient has advanced to a nasogastric feeding with a 75% solution of Meritine. To provide this, you should mix 250 ml of Meritine with _____ ml of water.

4. You have prepared 1,000 ml of a 50% solution of Ensure for a tube feeding. The physician changes the order to 1,000 ml of a 25% solution. You will need to add _____ ml of _____ to _____ ml of the 50% solution.

5. The physician orders 500 ml of a 1:4 Isocal solution for a jejunostomy feeding. You should use _____ ml of Isocal and _____ ml of water.

Topical solutions

The answers to these problems follow on page 181.

1. 60 ml of a 2% hydrogen peroxide solution for wound care contains _____ ml of peroxide.

2. To change the above 2% solution to a 1% solution, you need to add _____ .

3. To make a sodium hypochlorite soak of 500 ml of a 0.5% (V/V) solution, you must use _____ ml of sodium hypochlorite concentrate (100%) and _____ ml of diluent.

4. To prepare 500 ml of a 1:40,000 silver nitrate solution, you must use _____ ml of a 1:1,000 stock solution of silver nitrate and _____ ml of diluent.

5. To yield a 15% neomycin solution, you should add _____ G of neomycin powder to 1,000 ml of solution.

6. To prepare 1,000 ml of 1:6,000 potassium permanganate solution, you must add _____ mg of potassium permanganate powder to 1,000 ml of diluent.

7. To prepare a mouthwash of 4 oz of 1:20 sodium perborate, you would add _____ G of sodium perborate powder to _____ ml of finished solution.

8. To prepare 1,000 ml of a 1:400 cupric sulfate solution from a stock solution of 2.5% cupric sulfate, you would use _____ ml of stock solution and _____ ml of diluent.

ANSWERS TO PRACTICE PROBLEMS

Enteral solutions

1. 750 ml
2. 250 ml of Isocal and 250 ml of water
3. 83.3 ml or 83 ml
4. 500 ml of water to 500 ml of the 50% solution
5. 125 ml of Isocal and 375 ml of water

Topical solutions

1. 1.2 ml
2. 60 ml of water
3. 2.5 ml of sodium hypochlorite concentrate and 497.5 ml of diluent
4. 12.5 ml of silver nitrate stock solution and 487.5 ml of diluent
5. 150 G of neomycin powder
6. 0.167 mg of sodium permanganate powder
7. 6 G of sodium perborate powder added to 120 ml of finished solution
8. 100 ml of stock solution and 900 ml of diluent

OTHER CONSIDERATIONS

When performing dosage calculations for certain patients and certain drugs, you will need to be aware of some special considerations. This chapter describes the considerations required when calculating pediatric dosages based on the child's body weight and body-surface area, among other methods. The chapter also presents information on calculating pediatric fluid needs, reviews significant factors to consider for patients of all ages who require individualized doses, and concludes with a discussion of the special needs of geriatric patients.

PEDIATRIC DOSAGES

When caring for a pediatric patient, remember that a child is not simply a small adult. Although drug administration routes are the same for children and adults, safe dosage ranges can differ greatly. Pediatric dosages differ from those for adults because a child's immature body systems may be unable to handle certain drugs. For example, a child's volume of total body water is much higher than an adult's, and this affects drug distribution. The pharmacokinetics, pharmacodynamics, and pharmacotherapeutics of drugs differ in children, requiring special dosages.

To calculate pediatric drug dosages accurately, use the dosage per kilogram of body weight or body-surface area method. Other methods, based on the child's weight or age, are less accurate but may be used for rough estimates. Whichever method you use, you are professionally and legally responsible for checking the prescribed pediatric dosage to ensure that it falls within the safe dosage range.

Dosage per kilogram of body weight

Many pharmaceutical companies provide information about safe drug dosages for pediatric patients in milligrams per kilogram of body weight. Based on this information, you can determine the pediatric dosage by multiplying the child's body weight in kilograms by the milligrams of drug per kilogram. Most health care professionals consider this the most accurate method of determining pediatric drug dosages.

Here is an example: If the suggested pediatric dosage for a drug is 50 mg/kg/day, use the dosage per kilogram of body weight method to calculate how much drug to give an infant who weighs 9 kg:

$$50 \text{ mg:}1 \text{ kg} :: X \text{ mg:}9 \text{ kg}$$

$$1 \text{ kg} \times X \text{ mg} = 50 \text{ mg} \times 9 \text{ kg}$$

$$X = \frac{50 \text{ mg} \times 9 \text{ kg}}{1 \text{ kg}}$$

$$X = 450 \text{ mg (daily dose)}$$

Patient situations

1. A pediatrician orders calcium EDTA 50 mg/kg/day I.M., in divided doses every 8 hours. The drug is prepared as 200 mg/ml, and the child weighs 44 lb. What volume of drug will you administer at each dose?

■ Determine the child's weight in kilograms:

$$X \text{ kg:}44 \text{ lb} :: 1 \text{ kg:}2.2 \text{ lb}$$

$$X \text{ kg} \times 2.2 \text{ lb} = 1 \text{ kg} \times 44 \text{ lb}$$

$$X = \frac{44 \text{ kg}}{2.2}$$

$$X = 20 \text{ kg}$$

■ Calculate the amount of medication to administer daily:

$$\frac{X \text{ mg}}{20 \text{ kg}} = \frac{50 \text{ mg}}{1 \text{ kg}}$$

$$X \text{ mg} \times 1 \text{ kg} = 20 \text{ kg} \times 50 \text{ mg}$$

$$X = \frac{20 \text{ kg} \times 50 \text{ mg}}{1 \text{ kg}}$$

$$X = 1,000 \text{ mg}$$

■ Divide the daily dose by 3 to determine the dose you should administer every 8 hours:

$$\frac{X \text{ mg}}{1 \text{ dose}} = \frac{1,000 \text{ mg}}{3 \text{ doses}}$$

$$X = 333.3 \text{ or } 333 \text{ mg}$$

■ Calculate the volume of drug to administer at each dose:

$$\frac{X \text{ ml}}{333 \text{ mg}} = \frac{1 \text{ ml}}{200 \text{ mg}}$$

$$X \text{ ml} \times 200 \text{ mg} = 333 \text{ mg} \times 1 \text{ ml}$$

$$X = \frac{333 \text{ ml}}{200}$$

$$X = 1.67 \text{ or } 1.7 \text{ ml}$$

Thus, you should administer 1.7 ml of the drug at each dose.

2. A 22-lb child is to receive cefoxitin (Mefoxin) 100 mg/kg/day I.V. in divided doses every 6 hours. The drug is available in 1 G/10 ml vials. What volume of drug will you administer at each dose?

■ Determine the child's weight in kilograms:

$$X \text{ kg:22 lb} :: 1 \text{ kg:2.2 lb}$$

$$X \text{ kg} \times 2.2 \text{ lb} = 1 \text{ kg} \times 22 \text{ lb}$$

$$X = \frac{22 \text{ kg}}{2.2}$$

$$X = 10 \text{ kg}$$

■ Calculate the amount of medication to administer daily:

$$X \text{ mg:10 kg} :: 100 \text{ mg:1 kg}$$

$$X \text{ mg} \times 1 \text{ kg} = 100 \text{ mg} \times 10 \text{ kg}$$

$$X = 100 \text{ mg} \times 10$$

$$X = 1,000 \text{ mg}$$

■ Divide the daily dose by 4 to determine the dose you should administer every 6 hours:

$$\frac{X \text{ mg}}{1 \text{ dose}} = \frac{1,000 \text{ mg}}{4 \text{ doses}}$$

$$X = 250 \text{ mg or } 0.25 \text{ G}$$

■ Calculate the volume of drug to administer at each dose:

$$X \text{ ml}:0.25 \text{ G} :: 10 \text{ ml}:1 \text{ G}$$

$$X \text{ ml} \times 1 \text{ G} = 10 \text{ ml} \times 0.25 \text{ G}$$

$$X = 2.5 \text{ ml}$$

Thus, you should administer 2.5 ml of the drug at each dose.

3. A 55-lb child is to be started on phenytoin 5 mg/kg/day in two divided doses for 3 days, then placed on a maintenance dosage of 3 mg/kg/day. Phenytoin is available as a pediatric oral suspension of 30 mg/5 ml. What volume of drug will you administer at each dose for the first 3 days? As a maintenance dose?

■ Determine the child's weight in kilograms:

$$X \text{ kg}:55 \text{ lb} :: 1 \text{ kg}:2.2 \text{ lb}$$

$$X \text{ kg} \times 2.2 \text{ lb} = 1 \text{ kg} \times 55 \text{ lb}$$

$$X = \frac{55 \text{ kg}}{2.2}$$

$$X = 25 \text{ kg}$$

■ Calculate the amount of medication to administer each day for 3 days:

$$\frac{X \text{ mg}}{25 \text{ kg}} = \frac{5 \text{ mg}}{1 \text{ kg}}$$

$$X \text{ mg} \times 1 \text{ kg} = 25 \text{ kg} \times 5 \text{ mg}$$

$$X = \frac{25 \text{ kg} \times 5 \text{ mg}}{1 \text{ kg}}$$

$$X = 125 \text{ mg}$$

■ Divide the daily dosage by 2 to determine the dose you should administer every 12 hours:

$$\frac{X \text{ mg}}{1 \text{ dose}} = \frac{125 \text{ mg}}{2 \text{ doses}}$$

$$X = 62.5 \text{ or } 63 \text{ mg}$$

■ Calculate the volume of drug to administer at each dose:

$$\frac{X \text{ ml}}{63 \text{ mg}} = \frac{5 \text{ ml}}{30 \text{ mg}}$$

$$X \text{ ml} \times 30 \text{ mg} = 63 \text{ mg} \times 5 \text{ ml}$$

$$X = \frac{315 \text{ ml}}{30}$$

$$X = 10.5 \text{ ml}$$

Thus, you should administer 10.5 ml of phenytoin at each dose for the first 3 days. You would perform similar calculations to determine the maintenance dose, as shown here.

■ Calculate the amount of medication to administer each day as the maintenance dosage:

$$\frac{X \text{ mg}}{25 \text{ kg}} = \frac{3 \text{ mg}}{1 \text{ kg}}$$

$$X \text{ mg} \times 1 \text{ kg} = 25 \text{ kg} \times 3 \text{ mg}$$

$$X = \frac{75 \text{ mg}}{1}$$

$$X = 75 \text{ mg}$$

■ Calculate the volume of drug to administer at each dose:

$$\frac{X \text{ ml}}{75 \text{ mg}} = \frac{5 \text{ ml}}{30 \text{ mg}}$$

$$X \text{ ml} \times 30 \text{ mg} = 75 \text{ mg} \times 5 \text{ ml}$$

$$X = \frac{375 \text{ ml}}{30}$$

$$X = 12.5 \text{ ml}$$

Thus, you should administer 12.5 ml of phenytoin daily for the maintenance dose.

Body-surface area calculations

An accurate way to calculate safe pediatric dosages is by body-surface area (BSA). With this method, you must plot the patient's height and weight on a nomogram to determine the BSA in square meters (m^2). (See *Using a body-surface area nomogram* for details on how to use a nomogram.) Then you multiply the child's BSA by the suggested pediatric dosage given in mg/m^2. The following equation shows how:

$$\text{child's dose} = m^2 \text{ (child's BSA)} \times \frac{(\text{drug dose}) \text{ mg}}{1 \text{ m}^2}$$

This calculation method is often used to calculate safe adult and pediatric dosages for antineoplastic drugs, such as methotrexate and cytarabine.

When you need to calculate an approximate pediatric dose

USING A BODY-SURFACE AREA NOMOGRAM

When calculating the dosage of an extremely potent drug (or of a drug for a pediatric patient), you must first determine the patient's body-surface area (BSA). To do this, plot the patient's height and weight on the nomogram, and connect these two points with a straight line. The point where this line intersects the BSA scale is the patient's BSA in square meters (m^2). For example, suppose a patient is 160 cm tall and weighs 65 kg. A straight line connecting the height and weight intersects the middle scale at 1.75, indicating that the patient's BSA is 1.75 m^2.

For an average-size child, you can use the simplified nomogram below. This scale determines BSA based on the patient's weight alone.

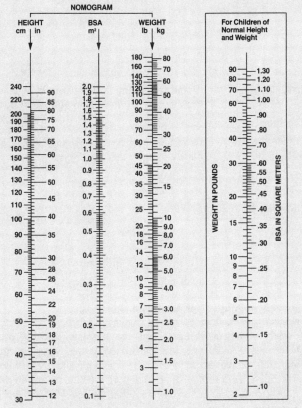

Reprinted with permission from Richard E. Behrman, ed. *Nelson Textbook of Pediatrics,* 14th ed. Philadelphia: W.B. Saunders Co., 1992.

based on an adult dose, the BSA method can help ensure accuracy. Use the child's BSA in the following equation:

$$\text{child's dose} = \frac{\text{child's BSA}}{\substack{\text{average adult BSA} \\ (1.73 \text{ m}^2)}} \times \text{average adult dose}$$

Patient situations

1. The suggested pediatric dosage of methotrexate is 3.3 mg/m². If a child is 35 in tall and weighs 60 lb, how much methotrexate should the child receive?

▪ Use the nomogram to determine that the BSA is 0.82 m².
▪ Use the child's BSA in the equation and solve for X:

$$X = 0.82 \text{ m}^2 \times \frac{3.3 \text{ mg}}{1 \text{ m}^2}$$

$$X = 2.7 \text{ mg}$$

Thus, the child should receive 2.7 mg of methotrexate.

2. A child is 41 in tall and weighs 30 lb. What would be a safe dose for this child if the average adult dose is 100 mg?

▪ Use the nomogram to determine that the child's BSA is 0.68 m².
▪ Divide the child's BSA by 1.73 m² (the average adult BSA), and multiply the result by the average adult dose:

$$X = \frac{0.68 \text{ m}^2}{1.73 \text{ m}^2} \times 100 \text{ mg}$$

▪ Solve for X:

$$X = \frac{68 \text{ mg}}{1.73}$$

$$X = 39.3 \text{ or } 39 \text{ mg}$$

Thus, the child should receive 39 mg of the drug.

Other calculations for pediatric dosages

To verify pediatric dosages, you can use one of three other calculations: Fried's rule, Clark's rule, or Young's rule. Because these rules derive the pediatric dose from an average adult dose and assume an average developmental level for a child, their results are only approximate. They can be used to help verify dosages, *not* to determine them.

Fried's rule

Based on the child's age only, Fried's rule usually is used to verify dosages for children under age 1.

$$\frac{\text{child's age (months)}}{150 \text{ months}} \times \text{average adult dose} = \text{child's dose}$$
(age at which an adult
dose would be appropriate)

The following example shows how to use this equation. The average adult dose of a drug is 125 mg. You need to determine the size of the dose for an 8-month-old child.

$$\frac{8 \text{ months}}{150 \text{ months}} \times 125 \text{ mg} = 6.66 \text{ mg (child's dose)}$$

Clark's rule

Based on body weight only, Clark's rule should be used for children over age 2. With this rule, the younger the child, the less accurate the dosage.

$$\frac{\text{child's weight (lb)}}{150 \text{ lb}} \times \text{average adult dose} = \text{child's dose}$$
(average adult weight)

The following example illustrates the use of this equation. The average adult dose of penicillin V potassium is 250 mg. You need to determine how much drug to administer to a 6-year-old child who weighs 68 lb:

$$\frac{68 \text{ lb}}{150 \text{ lb}} \times 250 \text{ mg} = 113 \text{ mg (child's dose)}$$

Young's rule

Based on the child's age only, Young's rule is usually used for children aged 2 to 12.

$$\frac{\text{child's age (years)}}{\text{child's age (years)} + 12} \times \text{average adult dose} = \text{child's dose}$$

This equation is used in the following example. The average adult dose of dicloxacillin is 250 mg. You need to determine how many milligrams to give to a 4-year-old child.

$$\frac{4 \text{ years}}{4 \text{ years} + 12} \times 250 \text{ mg} = 62.5 \text{ mg (child's dose)}$$

PEDIATRIC FLUID NEEDS

Infants and children have a greater need for water and are more vulnerable than adults to alterations in fluid and electrolyte balance. Because of the increased percentage of water in their extracellular fluid, children have a fluid exchange rate two to three times higher than that of adults and are, therefore, more susceptible to dehydration. Thus, determining and meeting the fluid needs of children is an important part of pediatric nursing. You can calculate the number of milliliters of fluid a child requires based on his weight in kilograms, metabolism (calories required), BSA in square meters, or age. Although results may vary slightly, depending on the method used, all methods are appropriate. (Note, however, that calculating fluid needs based on age is the least preferable method, because of the variability of size for any particular age.)

This section explains each approach to the calculation of maintenance fluid needs. Note that fluid replacement can be affected by clinical conditions that result in fluid retention or loss. Children with these conditions would receive fluids based on their particular needs.

Calculating fluid needs based on weight

A child weighing less than 10 kg requires 100 ml of fluid for every kilogram of body weight. To determine this child's fluid needs, follow these steps.

■ Convert the child's weight in pounds to kilograms:

$$\frac{\text{weight (lb)}}{2.2} = \text{weight (kg)}$$

■ Multiply the result by 100 ml/kg:

weight (kg) $\times$ 100 ml/kg = fluid requirements (ml/day)

A child weighing 10 to 20 kg requires 1,000 ml of fluid for the first 10 kg plus 50 ml for every kilogram above 10. To determine this child's fluid needs, follow these steps:

■ Convert the child's weight in pounds to kilograms, using the equation above.

▪ Assign 1,000 ml of fluid to the first 10 kg.

▪ Subtract 10 kg from the child's total weight, and multiply the remainder by 50 ml/kg:

(total kg − 10 kg) × 50 ml/kg = additional fluids needed

▪ Add this result to the base 1,000 ml. The total is the child's daily fluid requirement.

1,000 ml + additional fluids needed = fluid requirements (ml/day)

A child weighing more than 20 kg requires 1,500 ml of fluid for the first 20 kg plus 20 ml for every kilogram above 20. To determine this child's fluid needs, follow these steps:

▪ Convert the child's weight in pounds to kilograms, using the equation above.

▪ Assign 1,500 ml of fluid to the first 20 kg.

▪ Subtract 20 kg from the child's total weight, and multiply the remainder by 20 ml/kg:

(total kg − 20 kg) × 20 ml/kg = additional fluids needed

▪ Add this result to the base 1,500 ml. The total is the child's daily fluid requirement.

1,500 ml + additional fluids needed = fluid requirements (ml/day)

Calculating fluid needs based on calories of metabolism

You also can calculate fluid needs based on a child's caloric needs, since water is necessary to metabolize calories. A child should receive 120 ml of fluid for every 100 kcal (kilocalories) of metabolism. To calculate the fluid requirements, divide the child's calorie requirement by 100 (because the fluid requirements have been determined for every 100 kcal). Then multiply the result by 120 ml (the amount of fluid required for every 100 kcal), as shown in this equation:

$$\frac{\text{calorie requirements}}{100} \times 120 \text{ ml/kcal} = \text{fluid requirements (ml/day)}$$

Calculating fluid needs based on BSA

Another method for determining pediatric maintenance fluid requirements is based on the child's BSA. To determine the daily fluid needs of a child who is not dehydrated, multiply the child's BSA by 1,500, as shown in this equation:

BSA (m²) × 1,500 ml/day/m² = maintenance fluid requirements
(ml/day)

Calculating fluid needs based on age

A child under age 1 requires 125 to 150 ml per kilogram. To determine the lower boundary for the range of fluid needed, multiply the child's weight by 125 ml/kg. To determine the upper boundary of the range, multiply the child's weight by 150 ml/kg. The following equations illustrate this approach:

weight (kg) × 125 ml/kg = lower boundary (ml/day)

weight (kg) × 150 ml/kg = upper boundary (ml/day)

A child age 1 or older requires an initial 1,000 ml of fluid plus 100 ml for each year above 1 (not to exceed 2,500 ml/day). To determine the fluid needs of this child, then, you would follow these steps:

▪ Assign 1,000 ml of fluid for the first year.

▪ Subtract 1 year from the child's age, and multiply the remainder by 100 ml.

(Age − 1 year) × 100 ml = additional fluids required

▪ Add the result to the base 1,000 ml. The total is the child's daily fluid requirement.

1,000 ml + additional fluids required = fluid requirements (ml/day)

Patient situations

1. A child weighs 35.2 lb. How much fluid should be given over 24 hours to meet this child's maintenance needs?

▪ Determine the child's weight in kilograms:

$$X = \frac{35.2 \text{ lb}}{2.2}$$

$$X = 16 \text{ kg}$$

▪ Assign 1,000 ml of fluid for the first 10 kg.

▪ Subtract 10 kg from the child's weight, and multiply the remainder by 50 ml/kg.

$$X = (16 \text{ kg} - 10 \text{ kg}) \times 50 \text{ ml/kg}$$

$$X = 300 \text{ ml}$$

■ Add the result to the base 1,000 ml.

$$X = 1,000 \text{ ml} + 300 \text{ ml}$$
$$X = 1,300 \text{ ml}$$

Thus, the child should receive 1,300 ml over 24 hours.

2. A pediatric patient uses 1,000 calories per day. What are his daily fluid requirements?

■ Set up the equation:

$$X = \frac{1,000 \text{ kcal}}{100} \times 120 \text{ ml/kcal}$$

■ Solve for X:

$$X = 10 \text{ kcal} \times 120 \text{ ml/kcal}$$
$$X = 1,200 \text{ ml}$$

Thus, the patient requires 1,200 ml of fluid every 24 hours.

3. An infant has a BSA of 0.27 m². How much fluid does the infant require each day?

■ Set up the equation:

$$X = 0.27 \times 1,500 \text{ ml/day}$$

■ Solve for X:

$$X = 405 \text{ ml/day}$$

Thus, the infant should receive 405 ml of fluid each day.

4. A pediatric patient has a BSA of about 1.62 m². How much fluid does the patient require each day?

■ Set up the equation:

$$X = 1.62 \times 1,500 \text{ ml/day}$$

■ Solve for X:

$$X = 2,430 \text{ ml/day}$$

Thus, the child should receive 2,430 ml of fluid each day.

5. If your patient is 3 years old, how much fluid does she require each day?

■ Assign an initial 1,000 ml of fluid for the first year.

■ Subtract 1 year from the patient's age, and multiply the remainder by 100 ml.

$$X = (3 - 1) \times 100 \text{ ml}$$
$$X = 200 \text{ ml}$$

■ Add the result to the base 1,000 ml.

$$X = 1,000 \text{ ml} + 200 \text{ ml}$$
$$X = 1,200 \text{ ml}$$

Thus, the child requires 1,200 ml of fluid daily.

6. Your patient is 3 months old and weighs 4 kg. What is the appropriate range of fluid volume that should be administered to him?

■ To determine the lower boundary for the range of fluid that the patient should receive, set up the following equation:

$$X = 4 \text{ kg} \times 125 \text{ ml/kg}$$

■ Solve for X:

$$X = 500 \text{ ml}$$

■ To determine the upper boundary for the amount of fluid that the patient should receive, use the following equation:

$$X = 4 \text{ kg} \times 150 \text{ ml/kg}$$

■ Solve for X:

$$X = 700 \text{ ml}$$

Thus, the patient should receive 500 to 700 ml of fluid to meet maintenance fluid needs.

INDIVIDUALIZED DOSES

Some patients need unusually small or large doses. Others need doses calculated to the nearest milligram instead of the nearest 10 mg. For these special patients, the *exact* individualized dose and the correct dosage calculation can mean the difference between a drug underdose and an overdose.

Who are these special patients and why do they need such highly individualized drug doses? They are patients whose ability to absorb, distribute, metabolize, or excrete drugs differs from the norm. Some of them cannot absorb drugs from the GI tract because of upper GI disorders or surgery; deficiencies of gastric, pancreatic, or intestinal secretions; or passive congestion of GI blood vessels from severe congestive heart failure. These patients need drugs in parenteral form or in larger-than-average oral doses.

Patients with conditions that cause abnormal drug distribution from the GI tract or from parenteral sites to the sites of action also will need an altered dosing pattern. Premature infants and patients with low serum protein levels or severe liver or kidney disease cannot metabolize or excrete drugs as readily as normal patients and will require alterations in drug doses also.

You can help individualize drug regimens for most of these patients by assessing kidney or liver function, monitoring blood levels of drugs, and calculating exact doses, as needed.

Special needs related to weight

Take heed when determining drug dosages for an adult patient whose weight varies significantly from the average adult weight of 150 lb. For example, an 80-lb patient receiving an adult dose may experience toxic effects. Similarly, a 350-lb patient receiving an average adult dose will probably not experience the desired therapeutic response from the drug. If the physician orders the standard adult dose for a patient who weighs considerably more or less than 150 lb, you should question the order. To verify that the physician has ordered the correct dose, consult a drug reference for the correct dose in mg/kg/day. Then multiply this number by the patient's weight (in kilograms) to determine the correct daily dose.

Special considerations related to chemotherapy

Chemotherapeutic drugs used for malignant neoplasms also require special dosage calculations. Most chemotherapy is given in accordance with the patient's BSA, which is estimated by plotting the patient's height and weight on a nomogram (see "Body-surface area," pages 186 to 188). This method helps ensure that the patient achieves the desired blood concentration level of chemotherapeutic drugs. Thus, accurate recording of a patient's height and weight is essential throughout the course of chemotherapy.

Calculating dosages by BSA

With extremely potent or toxic drugs, such as antineoplastic agents, dosages are determined by BSA in square meters rather than by milligrams per kilogram of body weight.

Once you know a patient's BSA, you can use the ratio and proportion method to calculate the correct drug dosage. For example, suppose that a patient's BSA is 1.75 m², according to the nomogram, and that this patient is supposed to receive a drug dose of 1.6/mg/m². You could then use this information in a proportion to calculate the patient's dosage.

■ Set up the proportion:

$$1.6 \text{ mg}:1 \text{ m}^2 :: X \text{ mg}:1.75 \text{ m}^2$$

■ Solve for X:

$$1 \text{ m}^2 \times X \text{ mg} = 1.6 \text{ mg} \times 1.75 \text{ m}^2$$

$$X = \frac{1.6 \text{ mg} \times 1.75 \text{ m}^2}{1 \text{ m}^2}$$

$$X = 2.8 \text{ mg}$$

Patient situations

1. A patient with a BSA of 1.7 m² is to receive cisplatin I.V. every 3 to 4 weeks. The usual adult dose is 100 mg/m² every 3 to 4 weeks. What would be the safe and therapeutic dose for this patient?

■ Set up the proportion:

$$\frac{X \text{ mg}}{1.7 \text{ m}^2} = \frac{100 \text{ mg}}{1 \text{ m}^2}$$

■ Solve for X:

$$X \text{ mg} \times 1 \text{ m}^2 = 1.7 \text{ m}^2 \times 100 \text{ mg}$$

$$X = 170 \text{ mg}$$

Thus, the patient should receive 170 mg of cisplatin.

2. A patient with rectal cancer is to receive fluorouracil (5-FU) I.V. The patient's BSA is 1.82 m², and the recommended dose for rectal cancer is 1,000 mg/m² daily for 5 days each month. What would be the safe and therapeutic dose for this patient?

■ Set up the proportion:

$$\frac{X \text{ mg}}{1.82 \text{ m}^2} = \frac{1,000 \text{ mg}}{1 \text{ m}^2}$$

■ Solve for X:

$$X \text{ mg} \times 1 \text{ m}^2 = 1.82 \text{ m}^2 \times 1,000 \text{ mg}$$

$$X = 1,820 \text{ mg}$$

Thus, the patient should receive 1,820 mg, or 1.82 G, of fluorouracil daily for 5 days.

Special considerations for geriatric patients

A geriatric patient may require a drug dosage that differs from the usual adult dosage because of chronic illness or altered body weight. As a result, the physician usually determines the dose for each geriatric patient individually. And because each patient responds differently to aging and has a unique medical history, you must regularly and consistently assess each patient's response to drugs, whether or not he is receiving an average adult dose.

Nursing interventions

To help a geriatric patient comply with the medication regimen and avoid adverse reactions, follow these guidelines:

- Assess the patient's ability to obtain medications.
- Assess the patient's risk level.
- Simplify the medication schedule as much as possible.
- Educate the patient and family about the patient's medications.
- Encourage the patient to use a system of medication organization to ensure that he receives the ordered dosage.
- Help the patient to overcome cognitive and functional impairments.
- Help the patient to plan for follow-up medical care.
- Review medications periodically.

Altering tablets and capsules

When caring for a geriatric patient, you may want to crush the patient's tablets or capsules so that he can swallow them more easily. But first find out whether a liquid preparation of the same drug is available. If not, then determine whether crushing will affect the drug's action and follow these guidelines:

- Avoid crushing sustained-release (extended-time or controlled-release) drugs, although you may score and break some of them.
- Avoid crushing capsules that contain tiny beads of medication, although you may empty them into a beverage, pudding, or applesauce.
- Do not crush or score enteric-coated tablets, which usually appear shiny or candy-coated, because they are designed to prevent GI upset.

■ Avoid altering buccal and sublingual tablets.

If you need to crush a tablet, use a chewable form, which is easier to crush. Then use a mortar and pestle or a pill crusher, press the tablet between two spoons, or place it in a small plastic bag and crush it with a rolling pin. Once the tablet is crushed, give the patient a drink to wet the esophagus, and administer the tablet with more water as soon as possible after crushing. Unless contraindicated, you may mix the medication with pureed fruit.

If you need to break a tablet, use one that is scored. Be sure to use an instrument that will not harm you, such as a spatula or a single-edged razor blade. If the tablet is not scored, it should be crushed, weighed, and dispensed from the pharmacy, since you cannot be certain that you will break it into two even doses. You also should follow this procedure when breaking a tablet in smaller pieces than the score allows or when administering a portion of a capsule.

PRACTICE PROBLEMS

Pediatric dosages by body weight

The answers to these problems follow on pages 202 and 203.

1. The suggested dosage of tobramycin is 4 mg/kg/day for a neonate who weighs 3 kg. If the dosage must be divided and given every 12 hours, the child will receive _____ mg in each dose.

2. A physician orders 7.5 mg/kg of amikacin every 12 hours for a 4-kg infant. The child will receive _____ mg of the drug each day.

3. If the suggested dosage of pentobarbital is 1.4 mg/kg, you would give _____ mg to a 5-kg infant.

4. If the suggested dosage of phenytoin is 6 mg/kg/day, you would give _____ mg of the drug every 8 hours to a child who weighs 13 kg.

5. A drug order calls for 0.2 mg/kg/day of clonazepam for a child who weighs 16 kg. This child will receive _____ mg daily.

6. If the suggested dosage of chloramphenicol is 50 mg/kg/day in divided doses q 6 hours, you would give _____ mg to a 17-kg child with each dose.

7. If the suggested dosage of dimenhydrinate is 1.25 mg/kg, you would give _____ mg to a child who weighs 19.5 kg.

8. If a physician orders 25 mg/kg/day of nafcillin given in divided doses every 6 hours, you would administer _____ mg per dose to a 22-kg child.

9. A child who weighs 33 kg must receive a tetracycline injection. If the suggested dosage is 15 mg/kg/day divided into 2 doses, you would give _____ mg in each dose.

10. If the suggested dosage of thioridazine is 1.5 mg/kg/day, you would give _____ mg daily to a 16-kg child.

11. If the pediatric dosage of amikacin is 15 mg/kg/day, you would give _____ mg to a 6.5-kg infant every 12 hours.

12. If the pediatric dosage of clonazepam is 0.2 mg/kg/day, you would give _____ mg to a 27-kg child.

13. If the pediatric dosage of phenytoin suspension is 6 mg/kg/day, you would give _____ mg to a 21-kg child.

14. If the pediatric dosage of chloramphenicol injection is 50 mg/kg/day, you would give _____ mg to an 11-kg child every 6 hours.

15. If a child weighing 30 kg is to receive ampicillin 50 mg/kg/day, the total daily dose would be _____.

16. If a child weighs 25 kg and is to receive triamcinolone at a dosage of 2 mg/kg, you would administer _____.

17. If a drug order for a child weighing 22 lb calls for neomycin sulfate 50 mg/kg/day divided in four doses and the drug is available in 125 mg/5 ml, you would tell the mother to give _____ tsp each dose.

18. If a child weighs 44 lb and is to receive ampicillin at 100 mg/kg of body weight, the total daily dose will equal

_____.

19. If a safe daily dose of penicillin G is 100,000 units to 250,000 units/kg of body weight, a child weighing 20 kg could safely receive _____ to _____.

20. If a safe range of mezlocillin (Mezlin) is 100 to 300 mg/kg of body weight, a child weighing 40 kg could safely receive _____ mg to _____ mg.

Pediatric dosages by BSA

The answers to these problems follow on page 203.

1. A child who is 35 in tall and weighs 60 lb is to receive prednisone 60 mg/m^2 daily for 4 to 6 weeks until remission is achieved. The dose will be _____ mg based on a BSA of _____ m^2.

2. If the average adult dose of cytarabine is 350 mg daily for 5 days by continuous I.V. infusion, a child whose BSA is 0.9 m^2 might be expected to receive _____ mg daily.

3. If the average adult dose of doxorubicin is 100 mg I.V., a child with a BSA of 0.33 m^2 will require _____ mg.

4. A child who weighs 10 kg and is 70 cm tall is to receive lomustine 100 mg/m^2. The dose will be _____ mg.

5. A full-term infant weighing 7 lb is to receive an ordered dose of 25 mcg/kg of digoxin pediatric elixir. If the usual adult oral digitalizing dose is 0.5 to 0.75 mg, verify that the ordered infant dose is within safe limits, using the BSA method. The infant dose ordered equals _____ mcg; the safe range is _____ to _____ mcg.

Pediatric fluid calculations

The answers to these problems follow on page 203.

1. A 7-year-old child should receive _____ ml of fluid each day.

2. A child weighs 5.5 kg. He requires _____ ml of fluid to meet daily maintenance needs.

3. A 6-month-old girl weighs 6 kg. The girl should receive between _____ ml and _____ ml of fluid in 24 hours.

4. A child with a calorie requirement of 1,200 kcal/day needs _____ ml of fluid.

5. A child with a BSA of 0.45 m² requires _____ ml of fluid per day.

6. A 50-lb boy requires at least _____ ml of fluid per day.

7. A baby weighing 8 lb requires at least _____ ml of fluid per day.

8. A child's caloric requirement is 700 kcal/day. The child's maintenance fluid requirement is _____ ml/day.

9. A 14-year-old boy requires about _____ ml of fluid per day.

10. A child weighing 18 kg requires _____ ml of fluid per day.

11. A child has a BSA of 0.52 m². The child requires _____ ml to meet daily maintenance fluid requirements.

12. An 8-month-old boy weighs 16 lb. The boy should receive between _____ ml and _____ ml of fluid per day.

Chemotherapy calculations

The answers to these problems follow on page 203.

1. If a patient with a BSA of 1.4 m^2 is to receive 100 mg/m^2 of BCNU I.V. daily for 2 days, the total dose will be

_____.

2. If a patient whose BSA is 1.8 m^2 receives cisplatin 20 mg/m^2 I.V. daily for 5 days, the total dose will be

_____.

3. If a patient whose BSA is 1.5 m^2 is to receive 20 units/m^2 of bleomycin sulfate twice per week, to a total of 400 units, it will take _____ doses or _____ weeks to complete the treatment.

ANSWERS TO PRACTICE PROBLEMS

Pediatric dosages by body weight

1. 6 mg
2. 60 mg
3. 7 mg
4. 26 mg
5. 3.2 or 3 mg
6. 212.5 or 213 mg
7. 24.375 or 24 mg
8. 137.5 or 138 mg
9. 247.5 or 248 mg
10. 24 mg
11. 48.75 or 49 mg
12. 5.4 or 5 mg

13. 126 mg

14. 137.5 or 138 mg

15. 1,500 mg

16. 50 mg

17. 1 tsp

18. 2,000 mg

19. 2,000,000 units to 5,000,000 units

20. 4,000 mg to 12,000 mg

Pediatric dosages by BSA

1. 49.2 or 49 mg, based on a BSA of 0.82 m^2

2. 182 mg

3. 19 mg

4. 44 mg

5. 80 mcg; safe range is 64 mcg to 96 mcg

Pediatric fluid calculations

1. 1,600 ml

2. 550 ml

3. 750 ml to 900 ml

4. 1,440 ml

5. 675 ml

6. 1,554 ml

7. 363.6 or 364 ml

8. 840 ml

9. 2,300 ml

10. 1,400 ml

11. 780 ml

12. 909 ml to 1,090 ml

Chemotherapy calculations

1. 280 mg

2. 180 mg

3. 13 doses or 6.5 weeks

APPENDIX A

TEMPERATURE CONVERSIONS

When you need to convert a patient's body temperature from Fahrenheit (F) to centigrade (C) or vice versa, use the following conversion formulas.

To convert Fahrenheit to centigrade:

$$(°F - 32) \times \tfrac{5}{9} = °C$$

To convert centigrade to Fahrenheit:

$$(°C \times \tfrac{9}{5}) + 32 = °F$$

The following examples show how to perform these conversions. Suppose you need to convert a temperature of 102° F to centigrade. The formula would look like this:

$$(102° F - 32) \times \tfrac{5}{9} = °C$$
$$70 \times \tfrac{5}{9} = °C$$
$$\tfrac{350}{9} = °C$$
$$38.9 = °C$$

Suppose you need to convert a temperature of 35° C to Fahrenheit. The formula would look like this:

$$(35° C \times \tfrac{9}{5}) + 32 = °F$$
$$\tfrac{315}{5} + 32 = °F$$
$$63 + 32 = °F$$
$$95 = °F$$

APPENDIX B

DIMENSIONAL ANALYSIS

A variation of the ratio-and-proportion method used in this book, dimensional analysis (also known as factor analysis or factor labeling) is an alternative method of solving mathematical problems. Many nurses use dimensional analysis to calculate drug dosages because it eliminates the need to memorize formulas and requires only one equation to determine the answer. To compare the two methods at a glance, read the following problem and solutions.

The physician prescribes 0.25 g of streptomycin sulfate I.M. The vial reads 2 ml = 1 g. How many milliliters should you administer?

Dimensional analysis

$$\frac{0.25\ g}{1} \times \frac{2\ ml}{1\ g} = 0.5\ ml$$

Ratio and proportion

$$1\ g : 2\ ml \ :: \ 0.25\ g : X\ ml$$
$$X = 2 \times 0.25$$
$$X = 0.5\ ml$$

When using dimensional analysis, the problem solver arranges a series of ratios, called factors, in a single (although sometimes lengthy) fractional equation. Each factor, written as a fraction, consists of two quantities and their units of measurement that are related to each other in a given problem. For instance, if 1,000 ml of a drug should be administered over 8 hours, the relationship between 1,000 ml and 8 hours is expressed by the fraction

$$\frac{1,000\ ml}{8\ hours}$$

When a problem includes a quantity and its unit of measurement that are unrelated to any other factor in the problem, they serve as the numerator of the fraction, and 1 (implied) becomes the denominator.

Some mathematical problems contain all of the information needed to identify the factors, set up the equation, and find the solution. Other problems require the use of a conversion factor. Conversion factors are equivalents (for example, 1 g = 1,000 mg) that the nurse can memorize or obtain from a conversion chart. Because the two quantities and units of measurement are equivalent, they can serve as the numerator or the denominator; thus, the conversion factor 1 g = 1,000 mg can be written in fraction form as

$$\frac{1,000\ mg}{1\ g} \quad \text{or} \quad \frac{1\ g}{1,000\ mg}$$

DIMENSIONAL ANALYSIS *(continued)*

The factors given in the problem plus any conversion factors necessary to solve the problem are called *knowns*. The quantity of the answer, of course, is *unknown*. When setting up an equation in dimensional analysis, work backward, beginning with the unit of measurement of the answer. After plotting all the knowns, find the solution by following this sequence:

▶ Cancel similar quantities and units of measurement.
▶ Multiply the numerators.
▶ Multiply the denominators.
▶ Divide the numerator by the denominator.

Mastering dimensional analysis can take practice, but you may find your efforts well rewarded. To understand more fully how dimensional analysis works, review the following problem and the steps taken to solve it.

The physician prescribes X grains (gr) of a drug. The pharmacy supplies the drug in 300-mg tablets (tab). How many tablets should you administer?

▶ Write down the unit of measurement of the answer, followed by an "equal to" symbol ($=$).

$$tab =$$

▶ Search the problem for the quantity with the same unit of measurement (if one doesn't exist, use a conversion factor); place this in the numerator and its related quantity and unit of measurement in the denominator.

$$tab = \frac{1\ tab}{300\ mg}$$

▶ Separate the first factor from the next with a multiplication symbol ($\times$).

$$tab = \frac{1\ tab}{300\ mg} \times$$

▶ Place the unit of measurement of the denominator of the first factor in the numerator of the second factor; search the problem for the quantity with the same unit of measurement (if one doesn't exist, as in this example, use a conversion factor); place this in the numerator and its related quantity and unit of measurement in the denominator, and follow with a multiplication symbol. Repeat this step until all known factors are included in the equation.

$$tab = \frac{1\ tab}{300\ mg} \times \frac{60\ mg}{1\ gr} \times \frac{10\ gr}{1}$$

(continued)

DIMENSIONAL ANALYSIS *(continued)*

▶ Treat the equation as a large fraction. First, cancel similar units of measurement in the numerator and the denominator (what remains should be what you began with—the unit of measurement of the answer; if not, recheck your equation to find and correct the error). Next, multiply the numerators and then the denominators. Finally, divide the numerator by the denominator.

$$\text{tab} = \frac{1 \text{ tab}}{300 \text{ mg}} \times \frac{60 \text{ mg}}{1 \text{ gr}} \times \frac{10 \text{ gr}}{1}$$

$$= \frac{60 \times 10 \text{ tab}}{300}$$

$$= \frac{600 \text{ tab}}{300}$$

$$= 2 \text{ tablets}$$

For additional practice, study the following examples, which use dimensional analysis to solve various mathematical problems common to dosage calculations and drug administration.

1. *A patient weighs 140 lb. What is his weight in kilograms (kg)?*

Unit of measurement of the answer: kg

1st factor (conversion factor): $\dfrac{1 \text{ kg}}{2.2 \text{ lb}}$

2nd factor: $\dfrac{140 \text{ lb}}{1}$

$$\text{kg} = \frac{1 \text{ kg}}{2.2 \text{ lb}} \times 140 \text{ lb}$$

$$= \frac{140 \text{ kg}}{2.2}$$

$$= 63.6 \text{ kg}$$

2. *The physician prescribes 75 mg of a drug. The pharmacy stocks a multidose vial containing 100 mg/ml. How many milliliters should you administer?*

Unit of measurement of the answer: ml

1st factor: $\dfrac{1 \text{ ml}}{100 \text{ mg}}$

2nd factor: $\dfrac{75 \text{ mg}}{1}$

$$\text{ml} = \frac{1 \text{ ml}}{100 \text{ mg}} \times \frac{75 \text{ mg}}{1}$$

$$= \frac{75 \text{ ml}}{100}$$

$$= 0.75 \text{ ml}$$

DIMENSIONAL ANALYSIS *(continued)*

3. *The physician prescribes 1 teaspoon (tsp) of a cough elixir. The pharmacist sends up a bottle whose label reads* 1 ml = 50 mg. *How many milligrams should you administer?*

Unit of measurement of the answer: mg

$$\text{1st factor: } \frac{50 \text{ mg}}{1 \text{ ml}}$$

$$\text{2nd factor (conversion factor): } \frac{50 \text{ ml}}{1 \text{ tsp}}$$

$$\text{3rd factor: } \frac{1 \text{ tsp}}{1}$$

$$\text{mg} = \frac{50 \text{ mg}}{1 \text{ ml}} \times \frac{50 \text{ ml}}{1 \text{ tsp}} \times \frac{1 \text{ tsp}}{1}$$

$$= 50 \text{ mg} \times \frac{50}{1}$$

$$= 2,500 \text{ mg}$$

4. *The physician prescribes 1,000 ml of an I.V. solution to be administered over 8 hours. The I.V. tubing delivers 15 gtt/ml/minute. What is the infusion rate in gtt/minute?*

Unit of measurement of the answer: gtt/minute

$$\text{1st factor: } \frac{15 \text{ gtt}}{1 \text{ ml}}$$

$$\text{2nd factor: } \frac{1,000 \text{ ml}}{8 \text{ hours}}$$

$$\text{3rd factor (conversion factor): } \frac{1 \text{ hour}}{60 \text{ minutes}}$$

$$\text{gtt/minute} = \frac{15 \text{ gtt}}{1 \text{ ml}} \times \frac{1,000 \text{ ml}}{8 \text{ hours}} \times \frac{1 \text{ hour}}{60 \text{ minutes}}$$

$$= \frac{15 \text{ gtt} \times 1,000 \times 1}{8 \times 60 \text{ minutes}}$$

$$= \frac{15,000 \text{ gtt}}{480 \text{ minutes}}$$

$$= 31.3 \text{ or } 31 \text{ gtt/minute}$$

(continued)

DIMENSIONAL ANALYSIS *(continued)*

5. *The physician prescribes 10,000 units (U) of heparin added to 500 ml of 5% dextrose and water at 1,200 U/hour. How many drops per minute should you administer if the I.V. tubing delivers 10 gtt/ml?*

Unit of measurement of the answer: gtt/minute

$$\text{1st factor: } \frac{10 \text{ gtt}}{1 \text{ ml}}$$

$$\text{2nd factor: } \frac{500 \text{ ml}}{10,000 \text{ U}}$$

$$\text{3rd factor: } \frac{1,200 \text{ U}}{1 \text{ hour}}$$

$$\text{4th factor (conversion factor): } \frac{1 \text{ hour}}{60 \text{ minutes}}$$

$$\text{gtt/minute} = \frac{10 \text{ gtt}}{1 \text{ ml}} \times \frac{500 \text{ ml}}{10,000 \text{ U}} \times \frac{1,200 \text{ U}}{1 \text{ hour}} \times \frac{1 \text{ hour}}{60 \text{ minutes}}$$

$$= \frac{10 \times 500 \times 1,200 \text{ gtt}}{10,000 \times 60 \text{ minutes}}$$

$$= \frac{6,000,000 \text{ gtt}}{600,000 \text{ minutes}}$$

$$= 10 \text{ gtt/minute}$$

Reprinted with permission from Catherine M. Todd and Belle Erickson. *Dosage Calculations Manual*, 2nd ed. Springhouse, Pa.: Springhouse Corp., 1992.

REFERENCES

Baer, C., and Williams, B. *Clinical Pharmacology and Nursing,* 2nd ed. Springhouse, Pa.: Springhouse Corp., 1992.

Hudak, C.M., et al. *Critical Care Nursing: A Holistic Approach,* 5th ed. Philadelphia: J.B. Lippincott Co., 1990.

Luckmann, J., and Sorenson, K. *Medical-Surgical Nursing: A Psychophysiologic Approach,* 3rd ed. Philadelphia: W.B. Saunders, 1987.

Nursing94 Drug Handbook. Springhouse, Pa.: Springhouse Corp., 1994.

Olds, S., et al. *Maternal Newborn Nursing,* 4th ed. Menlo Park, Calif.: Addison-Wesley, 1992.

Olsen, J., et al. *Medical Dosage Calculations,* 5th ed. Redwood City, Calif.: Addison-Wesley Nursing, 1991.

Pickar, G. *Dosage Calculations,* 3rd ed. Albany, N.Y.: Delmar Publishers Inc., 1990.

Skidmore-Roth, L. *Mosby's Nursing Drug Reference, 1992.* St. Louis: Mosby Year Book, 1991.

Todd, C., and Erickson, B. *Dosage Calculations Manual,* 2nd ed. Springhouse, Pa.: Springhouse Corp., 1992.

Whaley, L., and Wong, D. *Essentials of Pediatric Nursing,* 3rd ed. St. Louis: Mosby Year Book, 1988.

INDEX

i refers to an illustration; t refers to a table.

i refers to an illustration; t refers to a table.

i refers to an illustration; t refers to a table.